Contemporary Neurology Series:

Fred Plum, M.D., and Fletcher H. McDowell, M.D./
Editors-in-Chief

Additional volumes in preparation

Dementia

Charles E. Wells, M.D. / Editor

 F. A. DAVIS COMPANY, PHILADELPHIA

Preface

Webster's Third New International Dictionary defines "dementia" [from the Latin *dement-, demens* (mad) $+$ *ia* (pathological consideration)] as "a condition of deteriorated mentality that is characterized by marked decline from the individual's former intellectual level and often by emotional apathy." As used today, dementia implies mental dysfunction due to organic disease. Dementia is thus contrasted with states of neural dysfunction not demonstrably due to organic brain disease, i.e., the so-called functional brain disorders. In common usage, it is further contrasted with states of acute organic brain dysfunction termed deliria or "acute brain syndromes."

This volume emphasizes mental dysfunction secondary to diffuse and progressive disease of the cerebral hemispheres in adult life. This focus on diseases that result in diffuse cerebral dysfunction in no way implies that the authors fail to recognize dementia as a frequent occurrence with focal brain disease; nor does it imply that the authors adhere to a particular theoretical position regarding the importance of focal versus global neural networks in the highest integrative functioning of man. Rather the focus here upon diffuse brain dysfunction reflects a recognition: (1) that equal attention to focal brain diseases and the resulting mental states here would necessitate a lengthy volume out of keeping with this monograph series, and (2) that focal brain disease is generally signaled by symptoms and signs of neural dysfunction other than or in addition to a simple decline in mentative capacities.

Even within the confines of diffuse brain disease, the authors make no claim that this volume is encyclopedic. Attention is paid here particularly to progressive disease processes. Much dementia (such as that resulting from an acute episode of cerebral hypoxia or hypoglycemia) is stable and non-progressive, even on occasion tending toward resolution, and these forms are neglected here. Primary amentia and mental disorders resulting from the progressive cerebral degenerative diseases of childhood are likewise beyond the scope of this monograph.

Dementia is a confluence where the neurologist, psychiatrist, psychologist, and the basic medical scientist meet. The published literature having to do with dementia in each of these related fields is enormous. To compile and catalog here all the information known about dementia might well adumbrate the topic. Rather we have sought to bring together authoritative treatments of a variety of related subjects dealing with dementia and diffuse brain disease. Some chapters deal with new and current topics; others, with extant materials organized anew to clarify this much neglected clinical condition. We hope the volume will not only illuminate various facets of our current knowledge but will equally emphasize the vast amount of work remaining to be done before we can pretend to understanding.

CHARLES E. WELLS, M.D.

Contributors

Stanley H. Appel, M.D.
Associate Professor of Medicine (Neurology) and Biochemistry;
Chief, Division of Neurology; Duke University School of Medicine

Ewald W. Busse, M.D.
J. P. Gibbon Professor and Chairman, Department of Psychiatry,
Duke University School of Medicine

Barry W. Festoff, M.D.
Postdoctoral Research Fellow, Laboratory of Neurobiology,
Duke University School of Medicine

Gunter R. Haase, M.D.
Professor and Chairman, Department of Neurology,
Temple University School of Medicine

Simon Horenstein, M.D.
Professor and Chief, Section of Neurology,
St. Louis University School of Medicine

William F. Meacham, M.D.
Clinical Professor and Chief, Division of Neurological Surgery,
Vanderbilt University School of Medicine

George W. Paulson, M.D.
Associate Professor of Neurology and Pediatrics,
Ohio State University College of Medicine

M. J. Short, M.D.
Assistant Professor of Psychiatry,
Duke University School of Medicine

Richard M. Torack, M.D.
Professor of Pathology and Anatomy,
Washington University School of Medicine

H. Shan Wang, M.B.
Assistant Professor of Psychiatry,
Duke University School of Medicine

Charles E. Wells, M.D.
Associate Professor of Psychiatry and Neurology,
Vanderbilt University School of Medicine

William P. Wilson, M.D.
Professor of Psychiatry,
Duke University School of Medicine

A. Byron Young, M.D.
Assistant Resident in Neurosurgery,
Vanderbilt University School of Medicine

Contents

Chapter 1

The Symptoms and Behavioral Manifestations of Dementia

Charles E. Wells, M.D.

Dementia comprises the spectrum of mental states resulting from disease of man's cerebral hemispheres in adult life. The American Psychiatric Association's *Diagnostic and Statistical Manual of Mental Disorders*[1] states that the organic brain syndromes (i.e., dementias) are manifested by the following clinical features: impairment of orientation; impairment of memory; impairment of all intellectual functions such as comprehension, calculation, knowledge, and learning; impairment of judgment; and lability and shallowness of affect. Dementia must be demarcated clinically, usually on the basis of symptoms and behavioral manifestations, from the acute brain syndromes (deliria) and those states of mental dysfunction not currently attributed to physical conditions (i.e., the functional disorders).

SYMPTOMATOLOGY

Defects in orientation, memory, intellectual functioning, judgment, and affectivity are stressed in the usual account of the symptomatology of dementia. These classic features may indeed dominate the clinical picture, but to focus exclusively on these symptoms is to emphasize the end states of the dementing process. Such an orientation neglects the richness of the clinical picture to be observed at its inception and in the earlier stages of the disease state before such gross malfunction is apparent. There is no question that if a patient presented himself to the neurologist or psychiatrist complaining chiefly of impaired memory and orientation, the first diagnostic consideration would be structural brain disease. Undue emphasis upon these features may, however, obfuscate the richness of the clinical symptomatology.

Early in the process of dementia a variety of other symptoms may present and may capture the attention of the patient, his family, and his physician. Many of these early symptoms of dementia differ little either qualitatively or quantitatively from those that occur in normal, healthy individuals who are exhausted, anxious, or subject to severe environmental pressures. These initial symptoms are particularly likely to involve impairment of those qualities that we believe are the result of whole brain function, of those qualities that we consider peculiarly human, perhaps of those qualities that we observe to be quite specific to the individual himself. Thus an early and frequent complaint is that the patient is "not himself," meaning that the patient and his companions have noted the onset of illness in terms of change in functions that are quite specific to the particular person, whether described in terms of alteration of drives, mood, enthusiasms, capacity to give and receive affection, creativity, or other features. Often there is a centering of the patient's attention on various somatic complaints, previously present or arising de novo, for which no adequate organic cause can be found and for which the usual remedies provide no relief. Here only the physician's acumen prompts him to search beneath the facade of somatic symptoms for the nidus of the problem.

2

Since it is often these most complex of human brain functions that are first affected in the dementing process, one might guess that usually the onset is readily discernible to the patient and to those about him, but this often is not the case. The onset is often dated in retrospect and with imprecision, the informant being aware that things are seriously amiss presently but unaware just when things began to move in this direction. The inability to date onset precisely attests to the effectiveness of the mental defense mechanisms working in the normal individual.

In perhaps the finest firsthand description of the onset and progression of the dementing process yet published, one observer wrote:[2]

Over the period that we worked together, . . . I became gradually aware that the fine edge of his intellect was becoming dulled. He was less clear in discussion and less quick to make the jump from a new piece of evidence to its possible significance. He spent more time over his work and achieved less; and he found it increasingly difficult to get his results ready for publication. He tended also to become portentious and solemn about his subject, as though one small corner of knowledge nearly filled his world, and the wider horizons were narrowing in. The change was so slow as to be barely perceptible, and the signs vanished when I tried to pin them down: they were like those faint stars which are seen more easily when they are not in the direct line of vision. I was left with a feeling of uneasiness which I could not justify.

. . . , after a period of absence, I looked forward with special pleasure to my homecoming, but when we met I knew with immediate certainty that I had lost the companion of my earlier years. The change was as yet mainly a loss of intellectual clarity and he remained himself, but a self that was subtly devitalised. To me it was as though a light had gone out, but no-one else seemed to notice anything amiss. . . .

By this time he was worried about his general health and attended a doctor from time to time with rather vague symptoms. For several years he had been said to have low blood-pressure, but nothing was found wrong apart from this, and he was reassured.

Wolff and Chapman[4,10] have studied extensively the changes in highest integrative functions which result from progressively larger focal lesions of the cerebral hemispheres in man. Although they did not study, serially, changes in function in patients suffering from progressive diffuse cerebral degenerative processes, it appears likely that the deterioration of function which they described with increasingly large focal hemispheric lesions reflects with fair accuracy the progressive dysfunction in the patient suffering from a diffuse cerebral deteriorative disorder.

Chapman and Wolff[4] delineated four categories of functions that are impaired in diseases of the cerebral hemispheres: (1) the capacity to express appropriate feelings and drives; (2) the capacity to employ mental mechanisms effectively for goal achievements (learning, memory, etc.) ; (3) the capacity to maintain appropriate thresholds and tolerance for frustration and failure, and to recover appropriately from them; (4) the capacity to employ effective and modulated defense reactions.

In the incipient phases of cerebral degeneration the individual experiences diminished energy and enthusiasm. He has less interest and concern for vocational, family, and social activities. Lability of affect is common often with considerable increase in the overall anxiety level, particularly as the individual becomes aware of his failing powers. He has less interest in goals and achievements, diminished creativity, less incentive to stick to a task, trouble concentrating, and difficulty screening out disturbing environmental stimuli. Failures, frustrations, changes, postponements, and troublesome decisions produce more annoyance and internal upheaval than usual, and it is harder to recover equilibrium after such disturbances. The individual's characteristic defense mechanisms are utilized more frequently and more blatantly, often with less than normal effectiveness.

As the disease progresses, the achievement of personal ambitions and fulfillment of social responsibilities become less important. The individual becomes increasingly absorbed with himself and his own problems and less concerned with the feelings and reactions of others. His anxiety increases and depression intensifies as he becomes increasingly aware of his diminished abilities; marked irritability with outbursts of anger may ensue. He has trouble making plans, dealing with new situations, and initiating activity. He avoids choices and decisions. Delayed recall and unreliability in calculations may be troublesome, as are slowed speech and understanding. Judgment suffers. Frustration tolerance is usually even further reduced. The person's characteristic defense reactions are further emphasized in his dealing with his environment, but they are less well regulated and less effective.

With worsening, drives and feelings diminish. The drive for achievement vanishes, and the patient may even lose interest in others' opinions of him. Appropriate dress and personal cleanliness may be ignored. There is usually a diminution of anxiety with progressive flattening of affect. Personal warmth and concern for others often disappear. Now the defects of function enumerated in the *Diagnostic and Statistical Manual*[1] become readily apparent. Defective memory, particularly for recent events, is blatant. Time and space orientation are faulty; the patient is easily lost. Learning ability is markedly impaired. The individual is unable to function in complex situations, has trouble understanding and following directions, and often loses the train of thought. Some patients are restless and overactive; others, lethargic and lacking in energy. Failure may now be ignored. With diminished drives and appetites, frustrations are not so likely to arise. The patient's characteristic premorbid defense mechanisms are now obvious, and reliance upon them may be damaging rather than protective. It is usually in this phase of disease that the motor and sensory neurological signs of brain dysfunction begin to appear. The appearance of specific neurological abnormalities does not depend so much upon duration of the disease process as upon the rapidity of the degenerative process and the extent and site of brain damage. Thus in rapidly progressive global diseases, signs of motor and sensory dysfunction may quickly assume prominence, whereas with more slowly progressive and more restricted

4

diseases, the traditional neurological examination may remain normal for long periods before definite abnormalities supervene.

As damage proceeds, drive and ambition disappear. The patient becomes apathetic. The human substance of the personality is lost. There is blunting of all feelings. Danger, loss, pain—even impending death—may rouse only the feeblest and briefest of responses. The patient now requires close care; he is grossly disoriented to place and time. Recent and remote memory are defective. Calculations are impossible save for a few sums long committed to memory. The patient is indifferent or unaware of people and situations. Perceptions are blurred and distorted. Frustrations may be hardly noted or not perceived, and defense mechanisms are dissolved. Survival provides opportunity for the appearance of paralysis, mutism, incontinence, stupor, and coma. Changes in level of consciousness are seldom conspicuous, however, until advanced stages of degeneration are reached, further contrasting the loss of highest-level functions with the preservation of lower-level functions. Neurological dysfunction is always impressive, however, in the terminal stages of hemispheric atrophy.

Thus early in the dementing process, the signs and symptoms of dementia are most related to the sphere of psychological dysfunction, and diagnosis can best be made on the basis of the psychiatric examination and psychological testing. With progression, the psychological functions further decline, but to them are added the neurological signs and symptoms of diffuse disease of the cerebral hemispheres. The division into psychological and neurological phases is perhaps theoretically inadmissible, but it serves to emphasize the utility of different diagnostic measures at different stages of the disease. No one with a modicum of medical and psychological knowledge fails to recognize the symptoms and signs of late-stage dementia; the symptoms and signs of early-stage dementia are, however, far from precise and predictive. The physician in such instances must be particularly alert, and perhaps particularly suspicious of organic brain disease if he is to avoid errors in diagnosis and therapy.

This account of the clinical pattern observed in dementia has stressed the variety and diversity of the clinical manifestations. Usually malfunction in varied spheres can be demonstrated by the time the patient with diffuse brain disease first seeks medical assistance. Such a mosaic of defects, formed from bits of dysfunction in multiple mentative capacities, is typical for the patient suffering from diffuse brain disease. In other patients, however, defects are limited to certain specific memory, language, recognition, or performance functions, with relative preservation of the spectrum of other mentative capacities. Such dense dysfunction in one area alongside good function in others is typically found in the patient with focal and circumscribed brain disease. Whenever one limited specific mentative defect alone is highlighted through careful and complete clinical evaluation, the likelihood that the dementia results from a single focal lesion is markedly increased. Of course certain defects, such as a profound aphasia, make appraisal of other mental functions difficult if not impossible to achieve, thus clouding the underlying issue. This topic is discussed at much greater length in Chapter 3.

DIFFERENTIAL DIAGNOSIS

Dementia must in particular be distinguished from the functional brain disorders and from delirium. Early in its course, the clinical picture of dementia may specifically suggest neurosis; later, functional psychosis or delirium.

The patient with mild to moderate brain disease often possesses features that suggest an anxiety neurosis or a depressive neurosis. Differentiation is usually possible on clinical grounds alone, though one may have to accept a sense of what is going wrong rather than obtain absolute proof early in the course of the disease. Thus before impairment of orientation, memory, and intellectual functions can be demonstrated with certainty, the examiner may respond to a vagueness in the presenting story, an imprecision in detail, or a lack of orderly thought processes that does not fit well with the patient's background and previous performance, bringing to mind the possibility of dementia. Other features are more specific. The neurotic patient almost never has impairment of orientation. Though he often complains of poor memory, its intactness can usually be demonstrated satisfactorily by persistent questioning. Similarly, though the neurotic patient often complains of impaired intellectual functions in general, when his cooperation is achieved for testing, this dysfunction can rarely be substantiated. Disorders of judgment and affectivity are conspicuous in both neurosis and dementia, though a different aura of dysfunction is noted in the two disorders. In neurosis, one senses usually that poor judgment is secondary to inner conflicts and emotions (particularly feelings such as anger and fear) that so preoccupy the individual and distort his perceptions that he is incapable of making logical dispassionate judgments. In dementia, poor judgment usually results from the individual's inability to attend to details and to assimilate the multiple factors that are usually weighed in decision-making, so that choice is directed on the basis of one particular bit of information with disregard for multiple other factors.

The nature of the affective change is also often a distinguishing feature. In neurosis, a pervasive feeling, such as anxiety or depression or anger, is likely to dominate the clinical picture, whereas in dementia the lability of affect is more striking. Thus, the demented patient appears in turn, and often with great rapidity, fearful then sad then angry, and in each situation the affectual response may be appropriate though excessive for the situation. This lability may not, however, be prominent early, when a pervasive feeling of sadness or fearfulness is not unusual.

With more severe disease, dementia is confused particularly with the functional psychoses (especially depression and schizophrenia) and with delirium. The differentiation of dementia from depressive psychosis, particularly in the aged patient, may be challenging. With a depressive illness, the history is often more precise and the date of onset more certain than is usual with dementing illnesses. Further, even though cooperation is hard to obtain and responses come with ponderous slowness, the examiner is usually able to demonstrate preservation of orientation, memory, and other intellectual functions in depressive illness — though their demonstration may demand unusual tenacity of the examiner. Certain biological features — such as anorexia, weight loss, constipation, early waking — are more typical of depression than of dementia. Again the mood in affective disorders is much more pervasive and less labile than in dementia. Although alteration in mood is common with dementia, differentiation from a primary disorder of mood is usually possible by clinical examination. From a practical standpoint, depressive illness more commonly mimics dementia than vice versa.

Although disorders of thought are prominent with dementia, it can usually be differentiated clinically from a primary disorder of thought, i.e., schizophrenia. When the cooperation of the schizophrenic patient can be obtained, preservation of orientation, memory, and intellectual functions is demonstrated in all save the most deteriorated of cases. Further, the disorder of thought seen in schizophrenia usually possesses a different texture from that seen in dementia. In schizophrenia one is struck by the sudden and inexplicable twists in the subject's thought content, the tolerance for conflicts, and the conclusions reached on logically unacceptable bases. In dementia, the thoughts expressed suggest more a meandering course—one can follow the progression of thoughts but it appears to lead nowhere. There is more a lack of identifiable objective and an inattention to detail than there are sudden switches in subject. Abnormalities of mood are, of course, also prominent in schizophrenia where one usually sees a flatness or inappropriateness of affect in contrast to the labile, perhaps poorly regulated but nevertheless appropriate, affective responses of dementia.

Delirium can usually be distinguished from the chronic dementing diseases on the basis of both history and examination. The history is usually one of abrupt and precise onset in delirium, whereas a stuttering or gradual course of uncertain onset is typical of dementia. Alterations in consciousness and physiological functions that are commonly present in delirium may allow an easy differentiation. Changes in level of consciousness are a hallmark of delirium; they are uncommon until the terminal phases of dementia. Depression of consciousness in delirium varies from an inattentive, dazed, dreamy state to stupor. Physiological alterations are both common and prominent in delirium—restlessness, tremor, slurred speech, insomnia, anorexia, nausea, vomiting, constipation, diarrhea, sweating, pallor, flushing, tachycardia, fever. While these may

7

be seen individually in dementia, they are seldom prominent and seldom dominate the clinical picture as they commonly do in delirium. The extreme variability of the clinical appearance, from moment to moment and hour to hour, should be emphasized in delirium—indeed, variability has been called the dominant feature of delirium—whereas a more level plane of dysfunction typifies dementia.

DISCUSSION

Dementia is defined as "the spectrum of mental states resulting from disease of man's cerebral hemispheres in adult life:" (1) to stress the absence of a single condition called dementia, and (2) to emphasize the concept of dementia as a broad continuum of dysfunction, ranging from a barely discernible deviation from normal to virtual cerebral death. The condition that we call dementia in any single patient at any one point in time is thus comparable to a single frame in moving picture film; it may catch the moment quite accurately and with good definition, but it gives only hints of what precedes and what follows. This very changing nature of the manifestations of diffuse and progressive brain disease makes it difficult for us to sculpture from the mass of our materials a form easily recognizable as "dementia."

Other than its changing appearance and character, there are multiple factors that make it difficult to crystallize the demented state conceptually. With focal lesions of the cerebral hemispheres, particularly those that involve primarily the motor and sensory pathways, we are often able to predict quite accurately the clinical state of the patient. Thus one can predict that a lesion properly situated within the left occipital pole will result in a right homonymous hemianopsia or that a lesion appropriately situated in the right internal capsule will result in a left hemiparesis and left hemisensory defect. With focal lesions located outside the primary motor and sensory regions, prediction of the resulting clinical state is much more difficult; with diffuse lesions such prediction of the resulting clinical state is virtually impossible, save with the most gross and totally destructive of lesions.

Dementia is difficult to approach clinically not only because of its panoramic nature and the lack of predictability in its symptoms and signs but because there is ample evidence that the severity of clinical dysfunction sometimes correlates poorly with the severity of the disease process as manifested pathologically. Although several studies [5, 7, 9] have indicated a fair degree of correlation between the severity of intellectual and functional deterioration and the severity of brain degeneration as demonstrated pathologically or by air contrast radiographic studies, there are still notable and intriguing exceptions. In one type of exception, the patient demonstrates profound dementia clinically, yet by conventional radiologic and pathological investigation, only moderate degree of brain atrophy. This may be explained by supposing that dysfunction secondary to organic factors precedes the actual brain atrophy by a predictable period — i.e., it may simply take a while for atrophy to be manifest. Thus more sensitive methods of examination (electron microscopy or perhaps special staining techniques for specific enzymes) might reveal structural defects; air contrast radiographic studies later might reveal progressive cortical atrophy; or longer survival might permit the occurrence of atrophy that might then be revealed by conventional pathological methods.

The more intriguing exception is the individual who appears to be functioning well mentally up until death but whose brain reveals severe atrophy on postmortem examination. Detailed premorbid studies of these individuals, who are usually remarked on only in passing in the literature or with incredulity at the postmortem examination, might be of great value in providing us clues as to what protects the individual with severe brain atrophy from the profound functional deterioration that we might expect to be its accompaniment.

In a general way, the ability of the individual to maintain socially acceptable function despite progressive brain degeneration has been attributed by various authors to the intellectual, social, vocational, and emotional resources prevailing before the onset of illness. This general thesis was promoted most persuasively by Rothschild[8] some years ago. He related the clinical dysfunction resulting from brain tissue loss to the individual's underlying "ability to compensate." He suggested, therefore, that the individual whose life had been marked by adaptability to changing events and circumstances would likely prove clinically resistant to the ravages of brain-cell death. This thesis has, unfortunately, never been thoroughly tested, though it has recently been echoed by Fisch and his associates[6] in a study of "chronic brain syndrome" in the aged population of the community. They found a few individuals with psychological evidence of rather severe brain damage who were able to live alone and still function in the community. They suggested that these individuals were able to do so "because of their superficial, strongly independent type of personality, their desire for autonomy, and their inability to tolerate caretaking persons or concepts of regimentation within an institution." Busse[3] has particularly stressed the relationship between socioeconomic status and the appearance of symptoms due to degenerative brain disease. Others [4, 10] have observed the functional deficit to be greater with rapidly progressive lesions than with slowly developing lesions of the same size. Thus we might guess that the clinical dysfunction from brain atrophy would be much greater should the final stage be reached over a period of several months than should the process have required several or many years. Despite these studies, we are left with a poor understanding why certain persons continue to function apparently well despite considerable brain atrophy whereas others manifest severe mental deterioration with apparently equivalent brain damage.

Another difficulty presents itself, particularly perhaps to the neurologist, in the conceptualization of the demented states. The neurologist is trained to deal with the brain as a complex of systems, and the conventional neurological examination is largely designed to evaluate the function of specific systemic functions, often teasing out with great subtlety dysfunction confined to one particular area of the nervous system or to a particular neural network. While certain particular forms of dementia (Korsakoff's psychosis, for example) result from well-localized or well-systematized lesions of the nervous system, much, and perhaps most, dementia reflects dysfunction of the brain as a whole. It is this concept—that of function and dysfunction of the brain as an entity—that often causes us the greatest difficulty. We must regard the brain as an organ if we are properly to evaluate its function, just as the cardiologist studies cardiac function as a whole and the nephrologist studies renal function as a whole. This does not imply that we must neglect study of component functions, for just as the cardiologist investigates vascular dynamics and muscular contractility, we may investigate modalities such as visual function and memory with great profit. This does imply, however, that the function of the brain as an organ is infinitely richer than what might be suspected from an investigation of its component systems individually. Thus both the conventional neurological approach to brain function (as a combination of sensory, motor, reflex, and symbol-manipulative functions) and the conventional psychiatric approach to brain function (as a combination of affectual, intellectual, and symbolic functions) are equally inadequate.

If we regard the peculiarly complex and creative activity of the human brain as the result of the workings of the highly developed cerebral hemispheres as an organ, whose function depends upon multiple morbid and premorbid characteristics, it follows that we must consider dementia as a peculiarly human disorder and that we can find no acceptable counterpart in nature for laboratory investigation. It is thus in these particularly human functions, which might truly be called the highest integrative functions, such as the capacity to think creatively, to deal effectively with new and complex problems, and to love and care for others, that the symptoms and behavioral manifestations of dementia may be most striking. The centrality of these functions for the human being makes dementia a worthy subject for our studies.

REFERENCES

1. AMERICAN PSYCHIATRIC ASSOCIATION: *Diagnostic and Statistical Manual of Mental Disorders,* ed. 2. American Psychiatric Association, Washington, D. C., 1968.

2. ANONYMOUS AUTHOR: *Death of a mind: A study in disintegration.* Lancet 1:1012, 1950.

3. BUSSE, E. W.: Brain syndromes associated with disturbances in metabolism, growth, and nutrition, in Freedman, A. M., and Kaplan, H. I. (eds.) : *Comprehensive Textbook of Psychiatry.* The Williams & Wilkins Co., Baltimore, 1967, pp. 726-740.

4. CHAPMAN, L. F., AND WOLFF, H. G.: *The cerebral hemispheres and the highest integrative functions of man.* Arch. Neurol. 1:357, 1959.

5. CORSELLIS, J. A. N.: *Mental Illness and the Ageing Brain.* Maudsley Monograph #9, Oxford University Press, Inc., London, 1962.

6. FISCH, M., GOLDFARB, A. I., SHAHINIAN, S. P., AND TURNER, H.: *Chronic brain syndrome in the community aged.* Arch. Gen. Psychiat. 18:739, 1968.

7. ROTH, M., TOMLINSON, B. E., AND BLESSED, G.: *Correlation between scores for dementia and counts of "senile plaques" in cerebral grey matter of elderly subjects.* Nature 209:109, 1966.

8. ROTHSCHILD, D.: *Pathologic changes in senile psychoses and their psychobiologic significance.* Amer. J. Psychiat. 93:757, 1937.

9. WILLANGER, R., THYGESEN, P., NIELSEN, R., AND PETERSEN, O.: *Intellectual impairment and cerebral atrophy: A psychological, neurological and radiological investigation.* Danish Med. Bull. 15:65, 1968.

10. WOLFF, H. G.: Dementia, in Beeson, P. B., and McDermott, W. (eds.): *Textbook of Medicine.* W. B. Saunders Company, Philadelphia, 1963, pp. 1569-1572.

Chapter 2

The Neurological Examination in Dementia

George W. Paulson, M.D.

This chapter suggests that special features characterize the neurological examination in dementia and hypothesizes that such features relate primarily to diffuse brain dysfunction. Certain signs that are not focal and do not indicate systemic disease will be emphasized. This approach does not imply that the neurological examination in patients who are demented is peculiar or difficult but emphasizes observations, common in dementia, that may be overlooked. In the demented patient, sensitivity to the environment may be changed, and rapidity and appropriateness of either local or total responses can be jeopardized. It is the total responses that are reviewed here. Answers to two questions are sought: In the patient whose history suggests but does not confirm a diagnosis of dementia, which observations might be particularly valuable to establish the presence of diffuse brain disease? In the patient known to be demented, which observations point toward diffuse rather than focal brain disease?

THE NEUROLOGICAL EXAMINATION OF THE AGED[16,34]

Despite youthful testimony to the contrary, advanced age is not synonymous with dementia. Many peculiarities of the elderly nervous system do not indicate loss of higher integrative function, although it is often difficult to separate the "normal" or common findings of aged patients from those that suggest disease. It is, of course, conceivable that many of the changes of aging, even the calm "wisdom of age," are secondary to loss of neuronal function. The fact that certain features seem inevitable, if one lives long enough, does not imply disease. Most observers have noted numerous degenerative changes that are common to advancing years regardless of whether aging represents a potentially avoidable disease or an entirely normal state. Loss of tissue elasticity, changes in nutrition, diminution of total blood flow, and frank insufficiency of both large and small blood vessels, plus other non-neurological phenomena—all can influence the neurological examination. In addition, the examiner must contend with both his own and the patient's psychological handicaps while evaluating an aged person. A feeble octogenarian with decreased hearing, slow motor responses, and a petulant unwillingness to be disturbed is not an ideal subject for extensive tests. The examination may be lengthened by the patient's general apathy, decrease in recent memory, and rumination on past events. It is therefore fortunate that many of the significant neurological manifestations of aging can be seen by purposeful observation alone. Awareness of these easily observable characteristics of age allows us to adopt a proper standard for normality while performing a neurological examination on a senile individual.

When an aged patient is first seen, it is commonly noted that gait is slow; and arm swing, head turning, and other associated movements are less conspicuous than in younger individuals. Moderate generalized stiffness, secondary to joint and ligament changes, and mild muscular hypertonicity are often observed.

The patient may be stooped, and he may relate his complaint in a quavering high-pitched voice that fatigues early in the interview. These changes of aging are so recognizable that actors tend to imitate parkinsonism when they wish to depict aging.

Examination of the eyes reveals a decreased ability or an unwillingness to converge, and upward gaze may be limited or sluggish. Miotic pupils are the rule, complicating evaluation of the light reflex. Funduscopic examination may show a waxy and indistinct disc, visualization of choroidal vessels, and diffuse granular pigmentation.[20,32,36,37] Elderly patients lose as much as 50 per cent of their sensitivity to both taste and smell. Hearing, particularly for high-pitched sound and background noise, is reduced. Tinnitus and vertigo may occur and be accentuated by positional change. The gag reflex is reduced, and this plus a decrease in the cough reflex leads to accumulation of secretions in the bronchial tree. In addition to mildly increased muscle tone and inconstant action tremors that are reminiscent of benign familial tremor, there may be slight generalized weakness of the muscles. Frank weakness is usually much less apparent than an overall decrease in quick coordinative functions. Muscular wasting, particularly in the calves and interossei, may be pronounced; and scattered fasciculations of the calves are often present.

The results of a carefully performed sensory examination can be normal, but decreased vibratory sensation at the ankles is almost the rule. Even though they are harder to measure quantitatively, pain and touch sensitivity are also somewhat reduced in many aged patients. The ankle jerks are often absent though reflexes in the upper extremities may be quite brisk. Abdominal reflexes, possibly because of a pendulous abdomen and lax muscles, may be hard to elicit. A pathological plantar response should not be observed, but the plantar response is often difficult to elicit in this age group, perhaps partially as a result of insensitivity of the sole and stiffness of the joints.

Numerous neurophysiological changes occur in normal aging, some of which are reflected in the clinical observation of aging patients.[40] Special studies of ocular function have included measure of latency of blinking, electroretinography, and electro-oculography. Electroencephalographers have written extensively regarding EEG changes, and changes in evoked responses in late life have been studied. Special interest of some groups has led to assessment of audiologic, olfactory, and gustatory function in the aged. Peripheral nerves have been assessed by time of conduction, study of the "H" reflex, and tests of peripheral end-organ sensitivity. Reflex responses and habituation change in age,[25,33] particularly the time required for transmission of some of the responses with longer reflex arcs. The threshold for ischemic pain is measurably different, as is the extent of nerve damage caused by ischemia.

Detailed review of these aspects of aging is not appropriate here, but some generalization is possible. Advanced age is associated with decreased rapidity of transmission, raised threshold, and relative insensitivity in almost all the phenomena mentioned above. The fatigability of response to stimulation is often increased and latency of response often prolonged as aging advances. Amplitude of response tends to diminish slightly in advanced years. Responses to drugs are modified, even distorted. Maturation from childhood to adulthood tends to stabilize neurophysiological responses, at a time when the flexibility and plasticity of childhood is lost. The transition to senility does not restore plasticity or flexibility, but is associated often with loss of neurophysiological stability and rapidity of response.

GAIT AND POSTURE IN DEMENTIA

Even the most superficial tour of institutions for chronically demented patients demonstrates that such individuals, young and old, walk in a clumsy or graceless fashion. Rocking movements of the trunk and neck, inappropriate associated gestures of the hands or similar "stereotypies," and a "slew-footed" and clumsy placement of the feet are particularly noticeable in younger demented patients. Myoclonic jerks or facial grimaces are characteristic of some of the progressive degenerative diseases, and athetoid posturing and tremors are seen with chronic or progressive diseases involving the basal ganglia.

Older patients, both those demented and those with normal intelligence, often have an unsteady gait that is marked by tremor of the hands and limbs. There is some tendency toward overall flexion, and though a rigorously upright posture is never typical of the average person, a military stance does not appear in late life unless in association with muscle spasm or low back pain. Associated movements of the hands during walking have not been specifically studied in elderly or demented patients, although in children with hemiplegia or with chronic diffuse brain damage the presence of associational patterns is more prominent than in normal children of the same age.[1]

Yakovlev[56] has discussed the tendency toward progressive changes in stance and station, including general body flexion, paratonic rigidity, and pelvicrural flexion contractures. He lists the following stages:

1. *The flexion attitude,* as mentioned, is typical of the aging patient in that he tends to sit or stand in a bent position with the neck slouched forward and hands cupped while the thumb is held in apposition to the forefingers. Such flexion tendencies are exaggerated when the patient walks, and if he is not warned as he starts rapidly, he may tend to tumble forward in a heap. If left to his own devices, spontaneous ambulation is infrequent and may be preceded by a "to-and-fro" inefficient foot shuffle— the "slipping clutch" gait often associated with arteriosclerotic brain damage. Some patients are incoordinated and ataxic of gait, and during their uncertain rambling they lean forward while grasping a side rail or touching a wall for support. Progressive dementia with increasing flexion may lead to a reluctance of the staff to get

the patient up in a chair, since he tends to curl forward and slump from the seat.

2. *Paratonic rigidity,* or *gegenhalten* ("opposition"), refers to the increased tone noted with passive manipulation of the limb, especially if the manipulation is done rapidly while the patient is urged to "relax, relax." Slow movements may avoid the resistance. "Involuntary rigidity," "perseveration," "postural fixation," "negativism," and similar phrases are used to describe this phenomenon. It is certain that some of the patients do attempt to cooperate, but to no avail. The inconstant rigidity is in contrast to the plastic rigidity of parkinsonism, which is usually best demonstrated in neck and shoulder groups, and must be distinguished from the spasticity due to activation of the stretch reflex as seen in the biceps or hamstrings of patients with corticospinal tract disease. Paratonic rigidity is frequent in dementia and usually becomes more obvious as cerebral deterioration progresses.

3. *Pelvicrural flexion contracture* is a much more striking phenomenon, and it is not at all rare when one surveys chronically bedridden patients in a demented and aged population.[17] A similar phenomenon is common in the late stages of progressive degenerative diseases in childhood and has been reported to follow repeated seizures.

As a rule seizures, myoclonic jerks, and other abnormal movements tend to diminish as pelvicrural contraction becomes permanent. In this position the knees are flexed toward the abdomen and the heels often rest against the

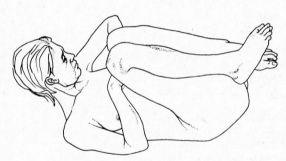

Figure 1. Pelvicrural contraction.

posterior thighs (Fig. 1). Although the ankle and knee jerks may be diminished, the hamstring reflexes are usually quite brisk. Even a gentle stimulus of the lower limbs may produce massive contractions of the proximal muscles which can be distinguished from the defensive reactions elicited with lower spinal cord disease. In the latter response, as in cord transection, the foot tends to contract and secondary movements occur higher in the limb, whereas with pelvicrural flexion the entire lower portion of the body contracts rapidly and inappropriately, with both limbs usually contracting at the same time.

REFLEXES

The Grasp Reflex

A distal moving contact in the palm may elicit flexion of the fingers, with grasping of the stimulating object (Fig. 2). When present, this response can be elicited in any position of the limbs and is not related to spasticity. In patients with more extensive brain lesions, the hand may not only clasp the stimulus but trap it as well or may pursue or grope after it in space. A firm stroking movement on the back of the hand may effect release. The variations and significance of the grasp reflex and grasping have been discussed at length during the past five decades.[2, 20, 47, 49]

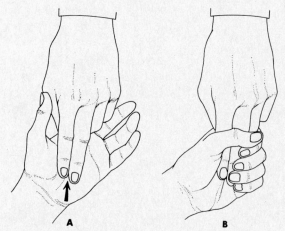

Figure 2. Grasp reflex. (A) Palmar stimulation; (B) grasp response.

The reflex may be predominantly a subcortical one, but most authors link the grasp reflex to frontal lobe disease even though lesions of the frontal lobe may either release or even abolish a prior grasp reflex. A grasp reflex has been observed in patients with frontal lobe tumors, and Bucy[14] has reported its presence with occipital lobe tumors as well. Vascular lesions and bilateral atrophic cortical disease are common associated disorders, and bilateral thalamic degeneration has been reported in association with this reflex. At one time it was stated that section of the corpus callosum plus destruction of one frontal lobe was sufficient to produce a grasp reflex, but neither uncomplicated section of the corpus callosum nor frontal lobotomy necessarily produces the reflex.[5, 53]

Probably as many as 20 per cent of aged and demented patients have a grasp reflex, and, in many, its presence reflects the severity of the disease as much as an exact localization to the frontal poles.[42] Although usually contralateral to the frontal lobe lesion, a grasp reflex can be present on either the ipsilateral or the contralateral side. When it appears on the ipsilateral side of a focal lesion, most writers invoke transitory diaschisis, acute cerebral edema, or extension of the lesion to the other side. It is also possible, of course, that such an appearance relates largely to a release phenomenon from the opposite frontal pole.

It has been suggested that the characteristic pointing position of normal humans, with the index finger extended and the others flexed into the palm, may have originated as an enfeebled or sublimated grasp reflex. Grünbaum[24] has noted preservation of what he calls the "pointing reflex" as an abnormal phenomenon in diffusely brain-damaged children. He reports that under favorable circumstances whenever the index finger is passively extended, the others tend to curl reflexly into the palm, at least until about age 2 to 3 years. This response is not easy to elicit in healthy adults, but might be expected to appear when brain damage is present. It may be similar to the traction response defined by Denny-Brown.[18]

The Tonic Foot Response

In 1938, Goldstein[23] discussed at length the tendency for the toes to turn down when the ball of the foot is stimulated (Fig. 3). The phenomenon is best elicited by direct pressure on the ball or sole of the foot, in contrast to the stroking necessary for a Babinski response. When a tonic foot response is present, the toes curl down in response to the stimulus, and there may be wrinkling of the skin of the sole, plus flexion and adduction movements of the toes.

The reflex has been associated with damage of the frontal lobe,[13] particularly its medial portions, and may represent a response related to the

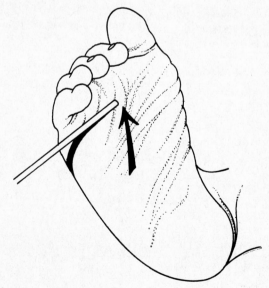

Figure 3. Tonic foot response.

"turning to" phenomenon of childhood. The tonic foot response may be similar to the palmar grasp; both these reflexes are almost always present in infancy but then disappear in normal adulthood.[21] In each instance a stimulus on the extensor portion of the hand or foot tends to counteract the grasping. It has been said that the presence of the tonic foot response on the homolateral side in a patient with brain tumor suggests either increased intracranial pressure or extension across the midline.

Oral Responses

Several reflex responses result from a stimulus applied to the mouth area. The best recognized are the snout and sucking reflexes. These are elicited by percussion (snout reflex) or stroking of the oral region (Fig. 4 and 5). Normal subjects manifest little or no response to such a stimulus. A positive response consists of a puckering movement as the orbicularis oris contracts. Some patients pucker and also turn toward the stimulus as if "rooting." Sucking and puckering movements occur via the nuclei of the fifth, seventh, and twelfth

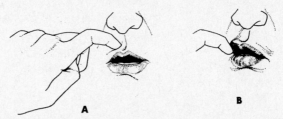

Figure 4. Snout reflex. (A) Puckering of lips in response to gentle percussion in the oral region; (B) Turning to a stroking stimulus in oral region.

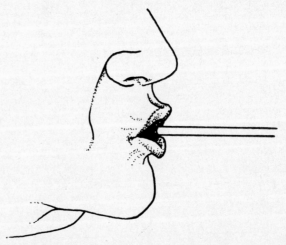

Figure 5. Sucking reflex, sucking movement of the lips in response to tactile stimulation in oral region.

cranial nerves, and some mouth movements are probably possible without dependence on any areas other than these low-level centers.[27, 28] Some patients with dementia show, particularly in the late stages of deterioration, not only incessant mouthing and licking movements but a persistent pursing of the lips that Darwin described many years ago.[45]

The snout and sucking responses, either or both, may be present in dementia; it seems unlikely that one implies a lower or a more severe lesion than the other. In general, a snout reflex in a person with delicate mouth muscles is of somewhat more significance than a sucking reflex. Normal individuals with powerful oral musculature may manifest fragments of these responses.

De Ajuriaguerra, Rego, and Rissot[4] attempted to quantify these oral responses and found that patients with severe Alzheimer's disease are particularly likely to show all types of the primitive mouth responses. In some patients the typical rooting reflex of infancy,[22] which consists of a turning toward the finger or tongue blade that has stroked the cheek, is also observed. The latter phenomenon suggests even more loss of normal inhibition than does a simple snout or sucking reflex produced by a stimulus at the lips.

Three major explanations are commonly offered for these oral phenomena: (1) A decline in overall levels of activation and awareness leads to movements that ordinarily would be inhibited.[51] (2) Specific localization has been postulated as a cause, particularly lesions between frontal cortex and globus pallidus, and bitemporal lesions. (3) The most commonly offered explanation is that these reflexes are ontogenetic or phylogenetic "release" phenomena: "Once a man, twice a child."

Some of the mouthing disorders seen in demented patients are not related to these reflexes and can be confusing. Any substantial group of old people is likely to include examples of lip-smacking and involuntary jaw movements, and a large and overactive tongue is commonly observed in edentulous patients. Reactions to certain drugs, such as phenothiazines, may cause buccolingual dyskinesia in senile patients.[41, 48]

Aside from the "tardive dyskinesias" and distinct from senile chorea and benign tremor, many involuntary mouth movements occur in aged patients that do not indicate any measurable decline in cortical function.

The Palmomental Reflex

The palmomental, or "palm-chin," reflex consists of unilateral contraction of the mentalis muscle when the thenar eminence of the ipsilateral hand is stimulated briskly (Fig. 6). Along with the common association of grasping and sucking,[10] this reflex is one of a series of phenomena that illustrate the neurological association of hand and mouth areas in early life.[39]

The palmomental reflex was originally described in adults with damage of the corticobulbar tracts.[11] One reason for the persistent interest in this somewhat inconsequential reflex is the long distance between the point of

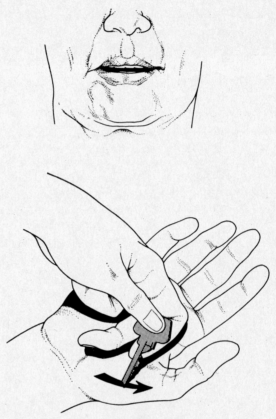

Figure 6. Palmomental reflex. (Below) Stimulation of thenar eminence; (Above) ipsilateral response of mentalis muscle.

stimulation and place of observation. As might be anticipated, it can be asymmetrical when there is facial weakness or an injury of the brachial plexus. The palmomental reflex is almost universally present in infancy but is usually absent or inconstant in normal adult life.[38] The reflex becomes more prominent with age, however, and is particularly common when severe dementia is present. It seems more common after a hemiplegic insult and is often noted in patients with parkinsonism or presenile dementia. Nevertheless, the presence or absence of this particular reflex does not predictably indicate either health or disease.

It is not clear why the wince-like movement associating a scratch of the palm and movements around the mouth is observed; it has been suggested that it might relate to the close representation of the mouth and thumb in the cerebrum, although the cerebral cortex is not required for its presence. Others have suggested a "short circuit" between the sensory and mouth areas. Bracha[12] suggested that palmomental reflexes may be an early sign of lesions of the frontal lobe, because he readily demonstrated the reflex in patients with a frontal tumor and after posterior frontal lobotomy.

In interpreting this reflex it should be emphasized that its reported frequency in normal individuals has varied depending on the observer and the technique used and that it is difficult to quantify.[36] It seems likely that many, even most, normal subjects have a weakly positive response if it is measured electrically, but in situations involving suprasegmental damage the reflex will be markedly exaggerated and persistent.

Corneomandibular Reflex and the Glabella Tap Relex

Although generally ignored by American neurologists, the corneomandibular reflex has been known for many decades. Wartenburg[54] emphasized it as a useful sign of supranuclear trigeminal involvement. It is best elicited by a firm stimulus (Wartenburg used a rounded glass rod), such as a cotton tip, applied quickly to the cornea. The strenuous blink is associated with a contralateral movement of the chin (Fig. 7). The mentalis muscle is likely

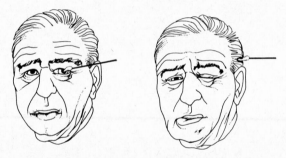

Figure 7. Corneomandibular reflex. (Left) Corneal stimulation; (Right) ipsilateral strong blink and contralateral movement of chin in response.

to move even when the complete chin movement does not occur. If the reflex is bilaterally present and both corneal areas are stimulated synchronously, then the chin moves forward. The corneomandibular response is an associated movement between the muscles innervated by the facial and by the trigeminal nerves. This "oculopterygoid" response relates directly to the forceful blink of the eye, and must be distinguished from numerous other facial synkinesias (as after Bell's palsy, when after partial recovery from damage to the facial nerve, the deep facial muscles contract jointly with the orbicularis oculi, or, when after partial recovery from an ocular motor palsy, there may be an associated movement between the levator palpebrae and the rectus internus). None of these latter facial synkinesias are related to the corneomandibular response.

Movements such as the corneomandibular response probably represent a dedifferentiation of an association that was present at earlier phases of development in the various muscles about the face. If this is true, then any state of heightened reflexivity may be expected to be associated with an overflow of facial movements from one area to another.

The corneomandibular reflex is often unilaterally present in patients with hemiplegia and is likely to be brisk and bilaterally present in patients with amyotrophic lateral sclerosis when the disease has extended rostral to the pons. It is also observed in patients with bilateral subcortical disease, as for example with lacunar infarcts. It has also been observed in patients with degenerative cerebral diseases, such as Alzheimer's disease. It can be postulated that the presence of this reflex is one more indication of diffuse brain disease. Wartenburg specifically stated that this reflex in its fully developed

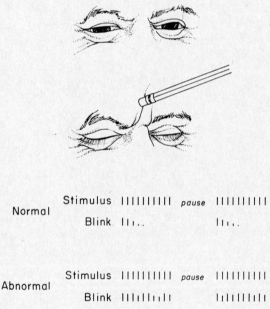

Normal	Stimulus |||||||||||	pause	|||||||||||
	Blink ||ı...		||ı..

Abnormal	Stimulus |||||||||||	pause	|||||||||||
	Blink ||||ı||ı||		|ı||||||ı||

Figure 8. Glabella tap reflex. (Above) Eyes at rest; (Below) response to stimulus.

form is not noted in normal persons. This is undoubtedly an extreme and inaccurate view, however, although the precise frequency of the reflex in normal patients remains unknown.

Light tapping over the glabella in a normal subject elicits reflex blinking, but with repetition the response quickly disappears. In many types of degenerative disease, but most particularly in parkinsonism, this glabella tap reflex may be accentuated and fail to fatigue (Fig. 8). The most striking feature[43] of the positive response is the absence of habituation on repeated testing. It seems likely that this primitive response, found by Minkowski in a 21.5-cm. fetus, would be present in other diseases in which cortical inhibition is diminished, or in which there are degenerative lesions in the basal ganglia.

In situations in which the level of cortical control is progressively diminishing, as in insulin-shock therapy, the reflex may be initially increased and then disappear.[31]

SOME GENERAL COMMENTS ON THE ONTOGENETIC APPROACH TO THESE REFLEXES

It is unlikely that a modern clinician would use the reflex responses discussed as a primary means of localization. Nevertheless, they retain interest and utility as monitors of central nervous system function, development, and deterioration. For example, the patient with an acute cerebral accident who gradually acquires an ipsilateral grasp reflex may be worsening because of brain swelling that involves both hemispheres. An elderly man with no clear evidence of intellectual deterioration may fall under suspicion, though not indictment, as having cortical atrophy if there is a prominent snout or sucking reflex. These reflexes are also of theoretical interest since the ontogenetic approach is a useful general explanation for most of them. It must be recognized that any single ontogenetic explanation represents interpretation through a narrow viewpoint, is overly simplified, and may inhibit anatomical explanations.

Coghill,[15] who viewed the central nervous system as a tool for maintaining the integrity of the individual, repeatedly emphasized the innate solidarity of the total organism. From his experience in Amblystoma he defined development as proceeding from the center to the periphery and originating from the innate developmental potentials of the organism. In 1929, he wrote, "During later periods processes of conduction in established tracts may be one activating factor in directing the line of growth, vascularization may be another. But, in the nerve cell as in the seed, growth as such must be regarded as the expression of an intrinsic potential of the cell." In addition to this spontaneous, dynamic view of growth, Coghill conceived development as a uniting of partial but discrete smaller patterns. Many embryonic responses can be interpreted in this fashion: that from general and broad patterns more precise and appropriate local responses appear.

The initial reaction to stimulation in amphibian and fish embryo consists of a contraction in a lateral plane, with partial or localized responses in later developmental phases. Hooker and his remarkably productive student, Tryphena Humphrey,[28] demonstrated that flexion is the first motor response in human embryos, and such flexion is an avoidance response. Extension of the embryo, perhaps having to do with postural and locomotor responses, is a later acquisition. Reflex "turning-toward" a stimulus generally appears later in fetal life than "turning-away." Throughout fetal life the intensity of the stimulus may affect the response and a seeking-after, or turning-toward, response can be converted into an equally intense turning-away if the stimulus becomes noxious.

25

Humphrey[27] has stated that the first reaction to stimulation of the oral area is simple mouth movement at 7 to 9 weeks in the human fetus. Sucking is a later and more complex phenomenon, and the common rooting reflex is quite variable in the fetus. Premature infants, and some term infants as well, have initial "confusion" and may display inappropriate turning-away or rejection movements while seeking the nipple.

Although it is tempting to feel that there is a regular and orderly progression of responses such as those listed by Humphrey,[29] and that skin responses, nociceptive sensitivity, smell, nerve conduction rates, and a host of other unrelated phenomena are explainable on the basis of an orderly progression from (1) more variable, inappropriate, slow, diffuse, to (2) more consistent, precise, rapid, and discrete responses—the situation is just not that simple. The pelvicrural response depicted in Figure 1 is somewhat like an embryonic flexion response, and the oral responses in dementia are similar to those of an infant. In the ontogenetic sense one assumes that rooting or grasping responses in demented patients indicate less severe disturbances than prominent rejection or apparent "hyperpathic" withdrawal, but such general conclusions are overstated.

Another concept similar to the ontogenetic one was offered by Thomson[52] in 1903 in an effort to explain associated movements. In certain clinical situations such as with basilar impression, after a cerebrovascular accident (particularly in childhood), or even as a benign family trait, subtle or obvious *mirror movements* mimic activity in the contralateral limb. When one hand contracts, so does the other. To some extent this phenomenon is part of daily experience—every school boy discovers how hard it is to pat his head and rub his stomach at the same time. Pursing of the lips or mouth movements are often associated with hand movements. Thomson stated that such associated movements, particularly flexion or extension movements of a lower limb when an upper limb is used, are explicable only in evolutionary terms. He also theorized that during normal development the constant presence of inhibitory influences leads to a gradual disuse of commissural fibers. More primitive creatures than man would retain more associated or combined movements. An alternative explanation would be that the more mature or trained commissural fibers themselves serve to inhibit the associated movements; it is not diminished, but perfected, connections that eliminate automatic associated responses.

The concept of higher levels serving as a damper to lower levels has been a prominent one in neurology for 60 years. Coghill's concept[15] of a patterned or predestined developmental template is attractive but incomplete. Modification, distortion, or development of normal interrelationships in the nervous system is directly dependent on the utilization, nutrition, and exercise of the central nervous system area involved. The ontogenetic and dynamic interpretation of growth has been enlarged by the additional emphasis on levels and mutual interaction.

In addition to his attention to the ontogenetic, evolutionary and anatom-icoclinical explanation, Denny-Brown[18] has been interested in what he has termed "positive" and "negative" phenomena. Although greatly oversimpli-fying his summations here, in general he linked positive aspects to frontal lobe disease and negative features to parietal lobe disease. The normal equilibrium may be disturbed, or there may be a predominance of either aspect. Frontal lobe lesions (positive) may lead to overreaction to natural visual or sensory stimuli, tactile automatisms such as grasp reflex, and per-haps such phenomena as preoccupation with the present and a loss of re-sponse to disagreeable situations. Parietal lesions (withdrawal) may be re-flected in primitive avoiding reactions, both visual and tactile, as well as in phenomena such as denial of disability, apathy, and anosognosia.

In addition to the primitive reflexes listed above there are many phe-nomena that are, to varying degrees, explicable by the jacksonian concept of a loss of higher levels, a de-escalation, or (in Jackson's words) a "dis-solution" that leads to release of phenomena that had been submerged or repressed since the earliest developmental phases. A few such phenomena are discussed below.

IMPERSISTENCE AND PERSEVERATION

Motor *impersistence* has been picked out of the large neurological reposi-tory of ignored observations by Miller Fisher.[19] Among the tests that can demonstrate this phenomenon are: (1) keeping eyes closed, (2) keeping tongue out, (3) maintaining fixation of gaze laterally, (4) persistence in a sound such as "ah" or "ee," (5) persistence of grip, and (6) combinations of these and others.

Although Fisher emphasized that motor impersistence is associated pre-dominantly with right parietal lesions, recent studies by Ben-Yishay and his colleagues[7, 8] suggest that motor impersistence correlates best with diffuse brain damage. Most neurologists would agree that although right parietal lesions are particularly likely to be correlated with this phenomenon,[9, 30] motor impersistence is also seen in many patients with diffuse dementia. One well-recognized example seen with bilateral cerebral disease is the difficulty patients with Huntington's chorea often have maintaining protrusion of the tongue. As a general rule, when a demented patient manifests marked motor impersistence, attention should be directed toward the right parietal lobe.

Perseveration, the repetitious performance of a motor or verbal action, has been associated with left inferior temporal and parietal lesions. The defi-nition has alternately broadened and narrowed in the last 50 years, and it is now clear that many different mechanisms can lead to what has been called perseveration. Severely demented patients, normal children, or even normal adults at times of extreme fatigue, may repetitiously rewrite a letter or per-form an act requested of them. When critical faculties are dulled, or if in-termediate memory is impaired, the same phrase may be uttered again and again. In one striking example, *transient global amnesia,* a phenomenon akin to perseveration is noted. In this condition patients seem unable to remember anything for longer than approximately 2 minutes, although distant memory and social actions are entirely normal.[50] During the brief period of illness, which usually consists only of hours or a few days, the patient may repeat the same phrase again and again, using slightly different words. The phenomenon is reminiscent of the repetition of stories by individuals who have forgotten that they have previously told them.

Allison and Hurwitz[3] studied perseveration in aphasia, which they distinguish from palilalia, recurrent utterances, stereotypes, and afterimages. They stressed the involuntary nature of perseveration and devised specific tests of verbal and motor performance that might elicit this response. Perseveration occurred in most aphasics, and might be one of the few residual indicators of a formerly severe aphasia after the general clouding of consciousness had disappeared. Although data suggest that either frontal or temporal lobes, particularly on the dominant side, are likely to be involved, a deeply placed midline lesion that disturbs the upper brainstem and interrupts subcortical connections was considered the most likely explanation for the perseveration in most cases.

APRAXIA

Although this chapter is designed chiefly to discuss generalized phenomena and although apraxia usually has more focal significance than impersistence or perseveration, persistent apraxia sometimes occurs in patients with diffuse and bilateral brain lesions and sometimes is absent in patients with focal brain lesions, regardless of the site. Von Monakow considered apraxia to be "an answer of the entire central nervous system to a massive regional or general insult."[35] There are localities of predilection, especially the entire territory supplied by the middle cerebral artery, particularly on the left. Although the local coloring of the apraxia may relate to the area involved, as predominantly motor or sensory, Brun and others have emphasized that lasting apraxia is usually associated with bilateral and diffuse disease.[55] Total disturbance of the left frontal or of the left inferior parietal area does not always result in apraxia, but severe damage of almost any region of the brain may result in a temporary apractic state. It has been suggested that each kinetic experience from childhood on leaves a complex engram that is superimposed on other engrams; it is thus not surprising that lesions of many areas may lead to perseveration of earlier and more rigidly formed or "instinctive" actions with loss of willed performance of the same act. For example, the apractic patient may be able to eat a meal placed in front of him but unable to imitate the eating of an imaginary meal.

Pick found typical apraxia in senile dementia, and others have noted its presence in presenile dementia, usually as a fairly late sign.

PSEUDOBULBAR PALSY

Diffuse bilateral subcortical and cortical disease of many causes can lead to pseudobulbar palsy. This phenomenon consists particularly of a loss of emotional control, usually as a brief, affectless crying with reddening of the face and wide-open mouth.[6] In rare patients the emotional incontinence is manifested as laughter. Spasticity of the oral or lingual areas with dysarthric speech is commonly observed. Swallowing may be limited, and salivation can be distressingly obvious. Atrophy of the tongue, as is seen with bulbar palsy, is not a feature. The syndrome is considered to represent supranuclear involvement with secondary brainstem release. The emotional incontinence of pseudobulbar palsy accompanies many conditions including bilateral strokes. It is particularly likely with small subcortical infarcts, and with multiple sclerosis. When a patient has dementia plus pseudobulbar palsy, severe bilateral cerebral disease can be assumed.

RESPIRATORY ABNORMALITIES

Among the numerous physiological alterations of aging is a change in response to carbon dioxide inhalation and to forced hyperventilation in the presence of diffuse brain disease. Patients with severe bilateral cortical disease appear overly responsive to the effect of carbon dioxide and may hyperventilate markedly on breathing air that has a high level of carbon dioxide.[26] On the other hand, apnea may be prolonged after voluntary overbreathing of room air as described by Plum and Posner.[46] The phenomenon of post-hyperventilation apnea (PHVA) can be tested by having patients take five deep in-and-out breaths, which lowers the arterial carbon dioxide tension transiently. Alert patients with normal brains rarely experience significant apnea, but subjects with brain damage often experience a period of apnea lasting 12 to 30 seconds or more. Both the excessive response to carbon dioxide and the prolonged posthyperventilation apnea may relate to loss of forebrain control. Neither of these phenomena has been extensively studied in dementia, but since they reflect diffuse cortical disease, abnormal responses might be expected.

Irregularities in respiration are as common in the very old as in the very young. Cheyne-Stokes respiration is particularly common in aged patients, especially in moments of drowsiness. This abnormality of rhythm does not have grave prognostic significance and is not known to correlate with dementia.

KLÜVER-BUCY SYNDROME

This syndrome is not properly discussed in a chapter that deals with non-focal neurological aspects of diffuse brain disease since traditionally the syndrome is observed after bitemporal lobectomy in monkeys. Pilleri[44] has stated, however, that a similar syndrome can develop with atrophic disorders such as Alzheimer's or Pick's disease. The major features include: (1) visual agnosia such that the animal seems unable to differentiate between living and nonliving objects; (2) oral behavior with licking and oral experimentation; (3) hypermetamorphosis, which implies a restless need to touch objects that are perceived; (4) decrease in emotional responsiveness, such as a loss of fear; (5) hypersexuality or pansexuality; and (6) changes in feeding patterns.

This rather rigid instinctive behavior is, according to Pilleri,[45] similar to the physiological repertory of normal infants. He suggests that lesions involve both the limbic and neocortical areas if the syndrome is evident in humans. Other authors have questioned the precise temporal localization of this syndrome. The full range of symptoms seen in monkeys and particularly the hypersexuality is not usually present in humans, but portions of the syndrome are quite common with Alzheimer's and Pick's disease.

SUMMARY

The thesis of this chapter is that the phenomena summarized, and others as well, relate primarily to the release of primitive activity when diffuse brain damage erodes cerebral inhibition. Anatomical correlations are always difficult when there are multiple lesions, but those that have been made have not offered a complete explanation of these phenomena.

To explain them phylogenetically is not completely adequate either but certainly does not build a wall against further investigations. Indeed such a concept points out the necessity to continue to search for other fetal or developmental responses in dementia, to assess the interrelationships between these reflexes, and to quantify the stimulus as well as the response. The prognostic value of these reflexes is not emphasized, because data on this point are not yet available. In the evaluation of dementia, as much as in any area of contemporary neurology, both specific observations and general principles await discovery.

REFERENCES

1. ABERCROMBIE, M. L. M., LINDON, R. L., AND TYSON, M. C.: *Associated movements in normal and physically handicapped children.* Develop. Med. Child Neurol. 6:573, 1964.

2. ADIE, W. J., AND CRITCHLEY, M.: *Forced grasping and groping.* Brain 50: 142, 1927.

3. ALLISON, R. S., AND HURWITZ, L. J.: *On perseveration in aphasics.* Brain 90:429, 1967.

4. AJURIAGUERRA, J. DE, REGO, A., AND RISSOT, R.: *Le réflexe oral et quelques activitiés orales dans les syndromes démentiels du grand âge.* L'Encéphale 52:189, 1963.

5. AKELAITES, A. J., RISTEEN, W. A., AND VAN WAGENEN, W. P.: *Studies on the corpus callosum. IX. Relationship of the grasp reflex to section of the corpus callosum.* Arch. Neurol. Psychiat. 49:820, 1943.

6. ARING, C. D.: *Supranuclear (pseudobulbar) palsy.* Arch. Int. Med. 115: 198, 1965.

7. BEN-YISHAY, Y., DILLER, L., GERSTMAN, L., AND HAAS, A.: *The relationship between impersistence, intellectual function and outcome of rehabilitation in patients with left hemiplegia.* Neurology 18:852, 1968.

8. BEN-YISHAY, Y., HAAS, A., AND DILLER, L.: *The effects of oxygen inhalation on motor impersistence in brain-damaged individuals: A double-blind study.* Neurology 17:1003, 1967.

9. BERLIN, L.: *Compulsive eye opening and associated phenomena.* Arch. Neurol. Psychiat. 73:597, 1955.

10. BIEBER, I.: *Grasping and sucking.* J. Nerv. Ment. Dis. 91:31, 1940.

11. BLAKE, J. R., AND KUNKLE, E. C.: *The palmomental reflex.* Arch. Neurol. Psychiat. 65:337, 1951.

12. BRACHA, S.: *The clinical value of the pollicomental reflex in neuropathology.* J. Nerv. Ment. Dis. 127:91, 1958.

13. BRAIN, W. R., AND CURRAN, R. D.: *The grasp-reflex of the foot.* Brain 55: 347, 1932.

14. BUCY, P. C.: *Reflex-grasping associated with tumors not involving the frontal lobes.* Brain 54:480, 1931.

15. COGHILL, G. E.: *Anatomy and the Problems of Behavior.* Cambridge University Press, New York, 1929.

16. CRITCHLEY, M.: *Neurologic changes in the aged.* J. Chronic Dis. 3:459, 1956.

17. DANIELS, L. E.: *Paraplegia in flexion.* Arch. Neurol. Psychiat. 43:736, 1940.

18. DENNY-BROWN, D.: *Positive and negative aspects of cerebral cortical functions.* N. Carolina Med. J. 17:295, 1956.

19. FISHER, M.: *Left hemiplegia and motor impersistence.* J. Nerv. Ment. Dis. 123:201, 1956.

20. FULTON, J. F., JACOBSEN, C. F., AND KENNARD, M. A.: *A note concerning the relation of the frontal lobes to posture and forced grasping in monkeys.* Brain 55:524, 1932.

21. GENTRY, E. F., AND ALDRICH, C. A.: *Toe reflexes in infancy.* Amer. J. Dis. Child. 76:389, 1948.

22. GENTRY, E. F., AND ALDRICH, C. A.: *Rooting reflex in newborn infants.* Amer. J. Dis. Child. 75:528, 1948.

23. GOLDSTEIN, K.: *The tonic foot response to stimulation of the sole: Its physiological significance and diagnostic value.* Brain 61:269, 1938.

24. GRÜNBAUM, A. A.: *The pointing position of the hand as a pathological and primitive reflex.* Brain 53:267, 1930.

25. HAGBARTH, K. E., AND KUGELBERG, E.: *Plasticity of the human abdominal skin reflex.* Brain 81:305, 1958.

26. HEYMAN, A., BIRCHFIELD, R. I., AND SIEKER, H. O.: *Effects of bilateral cerebral infarction on respiratory center sensitivity.* Neurology 8:694, 1958.

27. HUMPHREY, T.: *The development of mouth opening and related reflexes involving the oral area of human fetuses.* Ala. J. Med. Sciences 5: 126, 1968.

28. HUMPHREY, T.: *Embryology of the central nervous system: With some correlations with functional development.* Ala. J. Med. Sciences 1:60, 1964.

29. HUMPHREY, T.: *Some correlations between the appearance of human fetal reflexes and the development of the nervous system.* Prog. Brain Res. 4:93, 1964.

30. JOYNT, R. J., BENTON, A. L., AND FOGEL, M. L.: *Behavioral and pathological correlates of motor impersistence.* Neurology 12:876, 1962.

31. KINO, F. F.: *Nasopalpebral reflex: Application to neuropsychiatry, particularly to insulin shock treatment.* J. Ment. Sci. 95:143, 1949.

32. KORNZWEIG, A. L.: *Ocular conditions of the aged.* Geriatrics 19:24, 1964.

33. KUGELBERG, E., AND HAGBARTH, K. E.: *Spinal mechanisms of the abdominal and erector spinal skin reflexes.* Brain 81:290, 1958.

34. LOCKE, S.: *The neurological concomitants of aging.* Geriatrics 19:722, 1964.

35. MAYER-GROSS, W.: *Further observations on apraxia.* J. Ment. Sci. 82: 744, 1936.

36. McDONALD, J. K., KELLEY, J. J., BROCK, L. D., AND BARTUNEK, E. J.: *Variability of the palmomental reflex.* J. Nerv. Ment. Dis. 136:207, 1963.

37. OKUN, E., RUBIN, L. F., AND COLLINS, E. M.: *Retinal breaks in the senile dog eye.* Arch. Ophthal. 66:702, 1961.

38. OTOMO, E.: *The palmomental reflex in the aged.* Geriatrics 20:901, 1965.

39. PARMALEE, A. H.: *The palmomental reflex in premature infants.* Develop. Med. Child Neurol. 5:381, 1963.

40. PAULSON, G. W.: *Electrophysiologic Aspects of Development.* Unpublished monograph.

41. PAULSON, G. W.: *"Permanent" or complex dyskinesias in the aged.* Geriatrics 23:105, 1968.

42. PAULSON, G. W., AND GOTTLIEB, G.: *Developmental reflexes: The reappearance of foetal and neonatal reflexes in aged patients.* Brain 91:37, 1968.

43. PEARCE, J., AZIZ, H., AND GALLAGHER, J. C.: *Primitive reflex activity in primary and symptomatic parkinsonism.* J. Neurol. Neurosurg. Psychiat. 31:501, 1968.

44. PILLERI, G.: *The Klüver-Bucy syndrome in man.* Psychiat. Neurol. 152:65, 1966.

45. PILLERI, G.: *Schippenzeichen von Darwin "pursing of the lips" beim morbus Alzheimer.* Psychiat. Neurol. 152:301, 1966.

46. PLUM, F., AND POSNER, J. B.: *Diagnosis of Stupor and Coma*. F. A. Davis Co., Philadelphia, 1966.

47. RICHTER, C. P., AND PATERSON, A. S.: *On the pharmacology of the grasp reflex*. Brain 55:391, 1932.

48. SCHMIDT, W. R., AND JARCHO, W. W.: *Persistent dyskinesias following phenothiazine therapy*. Arch. Neurol. 14:369, 1966.

49. SEYFFARTH, H., AND DENNY-BROWN, D.: *The grasp reflex and the instinctive grasp reaction*. Brain 71:109, 1948.

50. SHUTTLEWORTH, E. C.: *The transient global amnesia syndrome*. Editorial. J.A.M.A. 198:778, 1966.

51. STERJILEVICH, S. M.: *La turbulence nocturne du vieillard psychotique*. L'Encéphale 51:238, 1962.

52. THOMSON, H. C.: *Associated movements in hemiplegia: Their origin and physiological significance*. Brain 26:514, 1903.

53. WALSHE, F. M. R.: *Syndrome of the premotor cortex*. Brain 58:49, 1935.

54. WARTENBURG, R.: *Winking-jaw phenomenon*. Arch. Neurol. Psychiat. 59:734, 1948.

55. WOLTMAN, H.: *Review of clinical and anatomical studies of apraxia, with special reference to papers by R. Brun*. Arch. Neurol. Psychiat. 10:344, 1923.

56. YAKOVLEV, P. I.: *Paraplegia in flexion of cerebral origin*. J. Neuropath. Exp. Neurol. 13:267, 1954.

Chapter 3

Amnestic, Agnosic, Apractic, and Aphasic Features in Dementing Illness

Simon Horenstein, M.D.

Analysis of the mental state of the demented patient with diffuse brain disease usually discloses specific amnestic, agnosic, apractic, and aphasic elements. The resulting disturbance, however, ordinarily exceeds their anticipated arithmetical sum. Study of these aspects provides the physician a degree of understanding of the neurological disorder, helps establish a viewpoint from which the patient may be managed and the family counseled, and affords valuable opportunities for studying mental mechanisms. Although each specific element may resemble corresponding deficits occurring in patients suffering well-localized, destructive lesions of the brain, the functional loss with diffuse brain disease is usually found to be milder, and, when combined with more general behavioral changes, problems of identification and interpretation frequently arise.

The presence of amnesia, agnosia, apraxia, or aphasia in dementia does not permit anatomical inference relative to localization of the disease, though rather general conclusions may be drawn concerning the texture of the morbid process.[8] Terms like *agnosic* or *apractic* dementia, moreover, do not necessarily imply that the whole disorder of behavior results from that particular feature dominating the mental state at the time of examination. When specific psychic dysfunctions derive from specific focal lesions the particular symptoms are likely to be more isolated and more severe than in diffuse disease. For example, the denial of illness and paranoid delusion that attend a gross defect in visual and somesthetic perception due to a focal lesion are, despite their severity, ordinarily not accompanied by other mental derangements. By contrast, behavioral and personality changes derived from the same kind of perceptual disorder due to diffuse brain disease are usually milder though associated with more global changes in mental function.

DISORDERS OF MEMORY

Some impairment of memory occurs in nearly every demented patient.[4, 61] In some cases the disorder is mild and attended by relative awareness with some degree of compensation. In others, amnesia may be intermittent or transient.[27] In a few cases memory loss dominates the clinical picture, and the demented state is attributable largely to the continuing disturbance of memory.[56] Amnesia is the central feature in such diverse conditions as Korsakoff's syndrome, certain posthypoxic and posthypoglycemic conditions, and instances of bilateral basal medial temporal lobe infarction.[14]

Postmortem examination of patients in whom persistent memory loss has been the major feature has generally disclosed bilateral cerebral lesions particularly along the walls and floor of the third ventricle or in the temporal lobe. The terminal segment of the columns of the fornix, mammillary bodies, anterior ventral nuclear complex, dorsomedial nucleus, and pulvinar of the thalamus are constantly affected in Korsakoff's syndrome. Bilateral lesions of these structures due to other causes also profoundly affect memory. The hippocampus, the medial basal portions of the temporal lobe including the hippocampal gyrus extending up to 8 cm. caudal to the temporal tip, or the cingulate gyrus may be involved instead. Affection of the amygdala and uncus appears not to alter memory. Most reported cases have bilateral though often asymmetrical lesions, suggesting that the functional system that serves memory is widespread, bilaterally organized, without internal anatomical specificity, highly redundant, and related to many diverse parts of the brain. Lesions become symptomatic only after attaining a significant mass while smaller ones may be effectively compensated. A few instances of severe memory disorder following unilateral temporal lobe resection have been reported, but the status of the residual temporal lobe was uncertain. The evidence is as yet incomplete that a unilateral temporal lobe lesion alone will produce a permanent memory defect.[12, 14, 56, 60]

The elements of memory are: (1) reception and registration of the material to be remembered (the memorandum); (2) organization and integration (retention); (3) recall of a stored memory into conscious awareness; and (4) reproduction of the memorandum. Each step may be deranged, but in most clinical cases of dementia simultaneous involvement of more than one element occurs.[60]

Reception and Registration

Reception and registration of the information to be remembered, the initial step in memory, depend upon the effectiveness of nonspecific mechanisms including attention, receptive language function, and perception. This initial step is readily disturbed by fatigue, emotional disorder, stupor, delirium, or metabolic imbalance. It represents the accession of information in proper temporal order and relationship. When the mechanisms of perception and registration are altered (as by a toxic delirium or a period of hypoxia), it may be extremely difficult to attract and retain the patient's attention long enough to present even a brief memorandum, or the memorandum may be altered in reception. Owing to restlessness, distractability, or inattentiveness during stupor, the patient may be unable to reproduce within a few seconds a memorandum as simple as the names of three common objects or for that matter the name of the hospital. With less disordered perception or registration, patients attend for longer periods and may be able to reproduce memoranda at longer intervals, but retention is impaired beyond that point. Competing stimuli such as noise or movement in the examining area may seriously compromise reception and registration in demented persons.

The period of registration without storage lasts from 3 to 5 seconds. Observations made on the duration and extent of memory loss for events prior to uncomplicated cerebral concussion indicate the minimal period of amnesia to be but a few seconds. It is inferred that the period of reception is followed by a short interval in which the memorandum may evoke responsive behavior; following this, the memorandum either disappears or is stored. The factors underlying the decision to store memories relate to the totality of mental function. The brief period in which the memorandum affects behavior and may be reproduced without being permanently retained is called the period of "scratch pad" or immediate memory.[23,24] A transient disturbance of scratch pad memory, as may occur in concussion or during an episode of cerebral hypoxia, need not interfere with other aspects of memory function. Once the concussed patient has recovered, new associations are formed and both old and new ones retained and recalled as well as ever.[48,49]

Defective registration may be incomplete. Many concussed patients retain memory fragments as fixed visual or auditory impressions but without temporal order or relationship, a portion of the memorandum being retained in a modified manner.[48,49]

Since much material to be remembered is received in the context of language or stored as a verbal memory, lesions of the left cerebral hemisphere, particularly the temporal lobe, may be associated with defective memory owing to impaired language reception. In such cases nonverbal memory, such as recognition of persons, may be spared. In other instances, especially when the right parietal or temporal region has been affected, the patient's recollection may reflect visual perceptual distortion. [12,45]

Reception and registration may be spared though other aspects of memory are severely affected. In the Korsakoff syndrome, for example, retention, recall, and reproduction are severely affected, while perception and registration are usually spared.[12,56] The patient is able to understand that he is to recall something and may be able to do so for several seconds, despite gross gaps in retention and recollection of more remote old and new experiences.

Perseveration may accompany disturbances of reception. This phenomenon, the repetition of a thought or act that is no longer appropriate, is frequently seen in patients with receptive language disorders. It is, however, far from specific and may be encountered in patients suffering diverse cerebral lesions. It may operate at a low level, such as a persistent motor response no longer appropriate to the command, or at a higher level, as by repetitive thoughts. Perseveration (or persistence of a memorandum otherwise destined for extinction) interrupts the perception and hence registration of sequential events.

Retention

Once perceived, the memorandum undergoes what may be thought of as storage or imprinting.[60,61] The process of retention[25] results in the formation of memory for temporal and spatial order and relationships that may be recalled at will and reproduced in some fashion. This organization and integration occurs without conscious effort. One is not ordinarily aware that he is storing and retaining memoranda, though storage may be facilitated by voluntary effort such as studying or attempting to memorize. Thus, what is stored is in part voluntary and a function of repetition.[14] Data from patients with head injuries suggest that the most recently formed memories are the most tenuous, for these are the ones most likely to be abolished when the period of retrograde amnesia extends beyond a few seconds.[48,49] It has been suggested by Russell[48] that recently formed memories require continual relearning to become well established, while older stable memories have already passed through this process.

Defective memory storage results in distortion of the memorandum, if it is recalled at all. Parts of a sequence are not remembered, or the serial relationship among a remembered number of items is incorrect. In mild memory disorder the internal arrangement of the memorandum is distorted. A patient asked to remember three common objects reproduces them correctly but with rearrangement. More severely affected patients fail to remember the objects, and what is remembered is out of order. Often the last part of the memorandum is recalled. The most severely affected patient remembers nothing. Mnemonic integration may occur in the presence of confusion or delirium, though the intense and horrifying, frequently repeated content of the mental disorder is more likely to be remembered than are the real events of the illness. In a condition like the Korsakoff syndrome, memory storage is subject to extreme impairment despite minimal disorder of perception, registration, and other mental functions. Other illnesses affecting the hippocampus, hippocampal gyrus, fornix, mammillary bodies, and anterior and dorsal median thalamic nuclei display similar deficiency of memory storage.[11,53]

Stored remote memories may normally undergo slow metamorphosis.[25,48] The relative intensity and temporal organization of their components become altered. This can readily be appreciated by testing one's own recollection of a remote and rarely recalled event against that of another who shared in it. The limits of such normal deterioration are variable within a relatively narrow range.

Memory storage beyond the stage of reception and registration is severely affected in most cases of dementia, resulting in loss of memory for current or ongoing day-to-day events, though old memories and skills may be retained.[45,56] In at least some of these cases loss of memory is relative, for some recent events may be retained, especially when emotionally charged.

Recall

Recall refers to the process by which previously stored memory is called into consciousness by voluntary effort or upon the provocation of an associated stimulus.[60,61] Defective recall does not usually exist without impaired retention. Most patients suffering disordered retention of memory display some degree of impaired recall of old memory beyond the limits of normal forgetting. Defective recollection is associated with loss of memory for events prior to the onset of the illness (retrograde amnesia) just as defective retention is associated with loss of memory for events occurring after the onset of the illness (antero-grade amnesia). The process of recall is susceptible to distracting forces such as fatigue, anxiety, or competition for attention.

Recall also is impaired by bilateral lesions of the hippocampus, hippocam-pal gyrus, fornix, mammillary body, parts of the thalamus, and the cingulate region.[12,14,27,56,60,61] The defect, however, is for memory of serial order among events in time and is not modality specific. The anatomical involvement thus appears to affect a system used in the transmission and retrieval of information stored elsewhere. Specific memories, such as the names of objects or their use, appear to depend upon other structures.[12,60] Complicated tasks such as reading, writing, and calculating may be little affected. The capacity to recall the con-secutive, sequential, and temporal relationships among prior experiences is impaired, ultimately to the point of leaving great gaps in memory or wiping out memory entirely. The evidence that recall ever totally escapes impairment in memory disorder is not convincing. In some cases recall of intermediate events (those of last week or last month) may be indistinct and those of years before so vivid that the patient believes himself living at that time, but when these recollections are tested against certain knowledge, they are usually found to be distorted.

Patients suffering disordered recollection with large gaps in consecutive memory may confabulate, particularly when they are unaware of the memory loss itself. Confabulation consists of the completion (or filling in) of defective recollection by the introduction or construction of a plausible but inappropri-ate item to complete the gap.[60] Some confabulations are thought to represent memory fragments, and others, incorrect associations leading to an account of an event that never happened. Confabulation may appear as a spontaneous declaration by the patient, who greets the examiner with the false recollection that he and the examiner had been talking but a few days ago about a mutually shared experience that never in fact occurred. When less conspicuous, confabu-lation does not occur spontaneously but may be provoked by asking the patient a concrete question the syntax of which presupposes certain knowledge. Asking whether he has been out of the hospital that day often provokes a confabulated reply, the implicit suggestion that he may not have been there all day stimu-lating the patient to spin a tale of going outside that has no truth. Confabula-tion has been regarded as functional, hysterical, an expression of denial of illness, and as mnemonic "completion" or compensation for memory loss of which the patient has some awareness. Victor[56] and others view it as an effort to "fill in" realized gaps in the continuity of experience. It is most severe when awareness of the memory loss is least precise and seems to depend on the pa-tient's inference that he should know an answer or the context of a situation. Its severity often reflects the abruptness and totality of the memory disorder. It is less common in slowly evolving conditions and more intense when the sensorium is disturbed.

Reproduction

Reproduction consists of conversion of the recollected material into an act that recreates it in a spoken, written, or enacted form with preservation of the orderly relationship of the memoranda.[25] Defective reproduction may be difficult to differentiate from defective recollection. Errors in reproduction may, however, be recognized by the patient who thus demonstrates the accuracy of his recall. Defects in language function impair the capacity to reproduce material, as stored memories are often recreated by verbal or language-based mechanisms.[45] In dementia, errors in reproduction and recall usually appear concurrently.

Behavioral Manifestations of Memory Loss

Amnestic states are often accompanied by grossly abnormal behavior, such as the confabulation just described. With failure of immediate retention, the patient fails to remember preceding events. The resulting gaps in continuing memory render him susceptible to disorientation in time and place as he can no longer focus on the very recent events of the last few minutes or hours. Severe memory loss may also be accompanied by restlessness and inattentiveness, the patients being attracted by unrelated, discontinuous, or novel events.[2]

When the patient is unaware of his amnesia, a paranoid reaction may ensue. This is not unique to memory disorder as most neuropsychological defects of which patients are unaware may be associated with paranoid reactions. An elderly person who has forgotten where he has left his spectacles may conclude that someone has hidden them. His memory gap is thus completed by an accusatory construct directed toward another person. Consequently, he may become angry, hostile, and physically abusive of others. At the same time, the patient, unaware of his memory loss, vigorously denies its existence. Clinical analysis invariably reveals defects in integration, recall, and reproduction simultaneously. The paranoid reaction is often used by the patient as a defense so that environmental attempts to compensate for his memory loss result only in further referential accusations. This pattern of memory loss is commonly encountered in senile and presenile dementia, frequently appearing as an exaggeration of premorbid reaction patterns.[4]

Awareness of memory loss is most likely when recall and reproduction are only moderately or mildly defective with perception and sensorium relatively preserved. One normally expects his store of memories to deteriorate, so that defective recollection with mildly impaired retrograde memory is less disturbing than is impairment of anterograde memory.[12,60] Impaired recollection for specific things, such as names of objects or the arrangement of a series, may be a manifestation of a developing disorder of language, especially when the left temporal or temporoparietal region is affected.[45,46,52] Some patients compensate for defective recall by learning to use facilitatory techniques such as reciting an alphabet mentally in an effort to find a letter that may then trigger recollection of the name of a forgotten person, place, or thing. Others use appointment reminders efficiently. Shopping lists, memorandum pads, or note-books used effectively minimize the handicap as long as the disorder remains stable. The language-based disorders of naming are usually compensated by paraphasia, the substitution of a word or phrase for that which cannot be retrieved and reproduced.[46,52,58]

The patient who is aware of his loss and unable to develop an effective com-pensatory device may become depressed. Depression is not a specific reaction to memory loss but may characterize any noncompensated loss of function or body part of which the patient is aware.[4] It is usually mild and rarely requires treatment.*

Continued recollection and reproduction of recently stored material are a feature of normal mental function. Such ongoing activity exerts an important influence on the quality of memory and determines its availability for recall and reuse.[48] An important result of this process is the ability to learn new or relearn old material. When recall and reproduction are defective, both new (anterograde) and older (retrograde) memory suffer. Novel associations are retained poorly and then only after particular difficulty in learning. Even though registration may be nearly normal, the inability to retain, recall, and reproduce results in serious learning impairment.

There are, then, two distinct forms of memory disorder that occur in de-mented patients. One is a defect in briefly held ("scratch pad") memory that results from impaired reception and registration of information destined to be discarded or stored for future use. The other defect involves retention, recall, and reproduction of previously learned, but, particularly, newly learned ma-terial. Neither form of memory disorder is disease-specific. Some degree of impaired reception and registration exists in most demented persons. In gen-eral, the more recent memories are most affected, but remote ones do not escape. The greater the degree of continuing anterograde deficit, the greater the disturbance of ongoing behavior and orientation.

AGNOSIA

Agnosia is the name applied to a group of disorders of recognition that occur when primary sensation is preserved.[13] Most agnosic patients display

---

*Stravinsky has described his own loss of recall rather pathetically: "I am pained, too, by sudden memory blanks; this is like waking at night in a foreign hotel and not knowing where you are. And my memory taunts me; while I may be unable to find the right address in it for an event of a month ago, and while yesterday is vague and last week might have evaporated, a great deal that was etched there three quarters of a century ago seems to lie on the tip of the tongue. These memory failures are more disturbing than reduced engine power, a car being able to run on one cylinder, after all, and a little low octane (not enough to flood the motor) so long as the transmission works and the chassis gets enough servicing." (Stravinsky, I.: *The New York Review of Books.* 12:8, p. 6, April 24, 1969.)

profound general changes in behavior, and the resulting difficulty in interpretation of test results has led to divergent theories of origin.[57,59] Gestalt psychology, maintaining that recognition depends upon perception against one's total background of experience and judgment (apperception), has occupied an important historical role in interpreting agnosic symptoms.[13] Many modern neuropsychologists view agnosic states as the result of defective temporal and spatial synthesis of information provided by specific primary sensory processes, combined with a general intellectual disturbance that interferes with the patient's ability to associate that which is perceived with previously formed mental images. As a result, though able to describe he is unable to recognize the nature of the stimulus presented.[3, 20, 21]

Agnosic disorders associated with widespread mental changes cannot be assigned focal significance with surety, though certain recognition defects may follow quite localized cerebral lesions.[8] Though one commonly speaks of agnosic states in modality-specific terms as *visual* or *object* or *somatic,* these conditions are often found together though differing in degree. Distinctive deficits of recognition may initiate or dominate the clinical state of the demented patient.[4] In degenerative illnesses these conditions usually evolve slowly and subtly, growing steadily worse with time (in sharp contrast to their gross and abrupt onset after cerebral infarction). Because of their relatively slow and symmetrical evolution in progressive dementia, recognition defects as such may not be detected until well established and then only after a conspicuous alteration of personality has occurred. When the dementing illness follows an acute focal disorder, cognitive function and behavior are often affected asymmetrically so that lateralized features bias the clinical state.[20,21]

Visual Agnosia

Visual agnosia presents a cluster of independent features often developing simultaneously and in parallel, including unawareness and hence denial of blindness, preserved appreciation of light, and impaired ocular movement, object recognition, and color discrimination. The patient is usually unable to select a figure from a background in which it is embedded or grasp the meaning of simple pictures. Visually agnosic patients are unable to read (but many patients who cannot read retain visual recognition). Hemianopia and visual inattention are not intrinsic to the agnosic disorder. Disorientation in visual space occurs early, the result of inability to recognize old configurations and learn new ones. Thus patients readily become lost in strange places when the agnosia is mild, and do so even in familiar surroundings when it is severe. Visual disorientation, i.e., inability to localize a point in space by sight alone, may further complicate the matter and enhance disorientation as concepts of distance become blurred. One visually agnosic patient, whose disorder resulted from hypoxia, stated that all the trees and houses on his street looked different from the way he remembered them and most looked alike, hence he could not find his way. As the defect in visual recognition becomes greater, particularly when combined with auditory and somesthetic agnosia, such familar places as the patient's own home become hopelessly confusing labyrinths.[1,2,6,9,10]

Concurrent with spatial disorientation, recognition of the nature or use of objects by sight alone becomes impaired. The patient cannot identify objects by looking at them though he is able to describe them. When other modes such as smell, taste, or touch are retained, recognition is achieved by their use. Some aspects of visual agnosia may be highly specific such as inability to recognize faces or colors though competence to identify objects by sight is retained.[2] A recent patient recognized his doctors and family only upon hearing their voices. In general, in visual agnosia common items of the same class, e.g., pencils, pens, crayons, cannot be readily distinguished from one another, and finally the general class cannot be identified by sight at all. The patient has become "mind blind" and without visual recognition.

Some disorder of constructional ability is present in most visually agnosic patients, a condition sometimes called *constructional apraxia*.[5,21] It is characterized by impaired ability to place objects in proper spatial relationship with one another or reproduce the relationship by copying. This disability includes the estimation of distance, so that the patient may be unable to reach toward and grasp objects by sight alone.[37]

Visual agnosia may be so complete that the patient has lost all appreciation of visual stimuli, responding only by withdrawal, startle, and pupillary reaction. He no longer recognizes that sight applies to him, behaving as though totally blind, yet failing to recognize his deficit.

Every agnosic patient, regardless of the modality involved, is incompletely aware of his deficit; hence, he neglects and denies it. The neglect, denial, and imperception are usually directly proportional to the severity of the defect. Though he may know that something is wrong, he cannot define it, and when he is most severely affected he does not even recognize that he is ill. He cannot, moreover, be taught the existence of his agnosia or informed of its meaning.[57,59] In such instances disordered registration prevents mnemonic integration and interferes with recollection and reproduction.[45] The patient may ascribe his difficulties to others and become paranoid, hostile, and accusatory. Having attained a degree of functional blindness without being aware of it, the visually agnosic patient denies it and behaves as though normally sighted. He walks into obstacles, fails to respond to edges and surfaces, and reaches inaccurately for doorknobs and light switches.

Physical examination of the visually agnosic patient usually discloses two conspicuous abnormalities—loss or impairment of facial expression and disordered ocular movements. Mimetic movements become infrequent, inappropriate, and finally disappear. Facial expression may convey bewilderment or surprise before becoming inexpressive and fixed. Loss of facial expression parallels lessening capacity to recognize faces and judge and discern events by sight. The resulting unnatural and meaningless facial expression announces the abnormality upon confrontation.

Disordered ocular movement is the second major physical sign encountered in patients with visual agnosia.[38,54] Gaze may be difficult to attract, being tonically fixed upon a small object. Patients often move their eyes in apparently random fashion though unable to do so on command. Thus, requests to look up, down, right, or left fail to result in appropriately directed movements though gaze may be attracted by a moving object. Many patients later fail to do even this, though gaze may then be attracted by sound or by touching a body part. Optokinetic nystagmus, attraction of gaze by stimulation in the visual field, exploration of space by sight, and visually induced placing responses become lost concurrently. Progressive disorders evolve toward total visual loss, but other conditions, e.g., hypoxia, may display maximal impairment at the beginning with slow recovery.[32]

Visual avoiding may be released so that sudden or gross movement toward the face produces involuntary withdrawal or retraction of the head, often leading to tonic neck extension. Visual avoiding is best tested with the patient seated and the head unsupported.[20]

Visual hallucinosis and paranoid reactions may accompany agnosic states, at times being highly complex and extending over long periods like dreams. They are usually treated as real, though accorded a degree of neglect similar to that applied to the visual loss itself. The content of the hallucinosis is variable. A patient may report that a large crowd of people walked back and forth in his room all night long and kept him awake. Other hallucinations may be vivid and grisly. Even so, they are described without the sense of terror usually encountered in drug-withdrawal delirium. Referential thinking may become severe as the agnosia extends to other modalities. Patients thus become suspicious of their families and attendants, believing that they have come under external control or persecution.[36]

A haberdasher who suffered Alzheimer's disease at 63 years of age exemplified the evolution of visual agnosia. His initial visual symptoms were inability to orient the knot of a tie within the slit of a shirt collar and to place gloves correctly in their boxes. He later became unable to shape men's hats and place them properly on customers' heads. He soon failed to recognize occasional but familiar customers and became lost on short walks. Eventually he could not locate by sight the examiner's finger when stationary in space though he could grasp it readily as soon as it moved. Finally he became functionally blind, remaining as unaware and incomprehending of the loss as he had been right along. At this point he collided with obstructions, failed to grope, and required guidance as he walked from place to place.

Somatic Agnosia

Agnosic manifestations, though modality-specific and divisible into visual or somatic ("tactile") forms for purposes of examination and interpretation, usually exist simultaneously and interact with one another, heavily contributing to the patient's mental disorder. Somatic agnosias are less obvious than visual and often remain undetected until they have become so gross that the patient cannot dress, owing to inability to orient clothing to his body. He may require help donning his coat, tying his shoes, or even putting on his spectacles. Though able to feel and describe what is in his hand, he is unable to recognize objects, textures, or differentiate weight by manipulation alone.[21] Inattentiveness to and unawareness of the state of his skin and body may result in his becoming dirty and unkempt. Abnormalities of posture and movement are evident on inspection. Postures and attitudes are fixedly maintained without rigidity.[19] Tactile avoiding, confusion about body side and finger identity, and inability to localize stimuli applied to the skin surface or recognize that he has been touched simultaneously in more than one place are common. Stimuli may seem more intense on the shoulder, face, or trunk than on the hand, fingers, or foot. When touched on the face and hand simultaneously, patients tend to be more responsive to the facial stimulus. This preference is best found when the eyes are closed but persists even after the patient has been shown the test.[23,31] Tonically flexed postures, relative immobility, and imperception or incomprehension of the meaning of multiple stimuli arising on the skin surface are accompanied by decreasing capacity to use implements, a condition called *ideational apraxia,* to be discussed later.

Gross focal lesions of one hemisphere may result in the patient's denying the existence of one side of his body, treating it as though it did not exist. Such patients are usually unable to dress, identify objects by form, name fingers, localize points on the body surface, attend to the affected side on bilateral simultaneous stimulation or to the hand when the face and hand of the same side are touched. Though maximal in the contralateral limbs, every one of these defects is represented to some degree on the limbs ipsilateral to the cerebral lesion even though sensation and perception are normal. This suggests that processes of cognition have bilateral significance even when the lesion is unilateral. Similarly, a gross unilateral visual perceptual lesion is accompanied by abnormalities of visual perception and recognition within the field ipsilateral to the cerebral lesion. These include disorders of construction and localization in space.[9,13,20,21,57,59]

Auditory Agnosia

Auditory agnosia[47] is common in demented patients though rarely sorted out for independent consideration. It may be seen in its most extreme form as acoustic asymboly. In this condition the patient has become deaf for all practical purposes. Customary psychic and orienting reactions to sound are absent. He attends to no sound and fails to recognize that ambient noises relate to him. Despite this gross deficit in auditory cognition, startle, audiogenic pupillary dilatation, and audiogenic myoclonus persist. There often appears to be a direct relationship between the degree of startle and the gnostic defect.

Looking at the sound source, its accurate localization, comprehension of spoken speech, recognition of sound, tones, tunes, and matching names with onomatopoeic words are impaired at less severe levels. Auditory agnosia may occur as a feature that can be isolated in dementia but is generally coupled with a corresponding degree of receptive language disorder. Auditory hallucinosis occurs and sometimes dominates the mental state. The patient just referred to developed impaired auditory function as his cortical blindness grew more severe. Early in his illness he could easily and accurately locate the source of sound by touch or ocular adversion though unable to find points by sight alone. He later became inattentive to spoken language, failed to understand ambient sounds such as that of a doorbell, misused words, and developed the delusion that a man called Harry was constantly talking to his wife. This false belief persisted until finally auditory and receptive language function virtually disappeared. He was then mute and his only response to loud sound was blink and startle.

SPECIAL CONSIDERATION OF THE CORPUS CALLOSUM[26]

Focal lesions of or near the corpus callosum may result in curious disturbances of mental function. Two situations associated with significant cognitive disorder involve the posterior part.[28,29,51] Lesions of the left hemisphere in or near the posterior or splenial portion may be associated with loss of the ability to read in the left visual field if the left cerebral hemisphere is dominant for reading. It results from interruption of projections from the right occipital and parietal lobes to the left posterior superior parietal lobe. If the patient suffers right homonymous hemianopia simultaneously he is totally unable to read though able to perform other visual tasks and to write.

More rostrally placed callosal lesions may spare reading but result in disordered use of the nondominant hand for naming by palpation or for recognizing letters or numerals written on the tips of the fingers of that hand. In order to name an object placed in the nondominant left hand, primary sensory information is projected to the right brain, where it is received and undergoes perceptual analysis, which permits description of its shape, weight, and texture. The information obtained from manipulation of the object must be received within a fixed temporal interval if it is to have meaning related to form. Perceptual integration in the right brain does not permit conversion of the information into a name or verbal description. This is usually a left temporoparietal function and the perceptual information must be transmitted to that side if it is to be named. The information projected to the left temporoparietal region is processed, a name selected, and this information projected rostrally to the left frontal lobe before a word is utttered which

47

names the object. In the absence of this mechanism the object may be described only as something, but may be recognized by sight or touch. Thus, memory and intermodal associations may be normal in the absence of naming, and other interhemispheric functions intact though certain transcallosal language functions have been lost.

APRAXIA

Apraxia is a general term used to describe inability to perform purposive movements though power, sensation, and coordination are preserved. Like visual and somatic agnosia it usually involves both sides except when it appears in the special context of a callosal or paracallosal lesion.[18,29,30,33]

Ideational Apraxia

Apraxia may be thought of in three distinct clinical forms. The first is an ideational disorder, called ideational or ideatory apraxia. The patient suffering ideational apraxia is unable to execute a command. He may do nothing, do something entirely different, or enact a distorted or disordered fragment. He appears to have forgotten how to perform the required act or to have lost the capacity to arrange properly the critical temporal sequences and spatial concurrences underlying the required movement, thus producing something new, unpredictable, and inadequate. When asked to make a fist he may stare at his hand, salute, or protrude his tongue. He may recognize the nature and describe the use of utensils though unable to hold them correctly or use them as intended. Thus, he may identify a pencil and describe its purpose but hold it improperly or use the eraser for writing. Ideationally apractic patients are generally unaware of their disability. As in other disease states compounded by unawareness (anosognosia), paranoid symptoms may be present. The patient with ideational apraxia is recognized by observing his attempts to use utensils or his performance of a fixed task with or without implements. He does not complain of that of which he is unaware, and he cannot be commanded to demonstrate his apraxia, rather doing so by his performance failures and his inability to describe in words how he should execute the required act. Echopraxia, compulsive imitation of movements, is common in ideational apraxia. Ideational apraxia frequently occurs in patients suffering focal lesions of the lateral and posterior parietal portion of the dominant cerebral hemisphere; it may be associated with a language disorder marked by echolalia and syntactical aphasia. It is also present in cases of widespread cerebral disease without conspicuous aphasia, though language function may be abnormal. Presumably the extensive disorganization of brain function in such cases causes decompensation of the elements underlying formation of the concept of progressive movements. Such conceptualization appears related to the dominant parietal lobe.[29,30]

Ideomotor Apraxia

Ideomotor apraxia is a conduction disorder. While ideational defects may be present, the unique feature is loss or impairment of the ability to imitate an act such as waving or saluting, despite comprehension of the task and ability to use the limb. It depends upon a lesion in the white matter of the dominant parietal lobe. This condition is often associated with conduction aphasia. The patient may be aware of his plight, often shaking his head and smiling quizzically as he realizes his error. Echopraxia is absent. Thus, the patient suffering ideational apraxia without aphasia knows that he is to do something but cannot recall or describe how to do it, and either substitutes another movement or does nothing. At the same time he may imitate compulsively. In ideomotor apraxia without aphasia, recall and verbal description are preserved but conduction from concept to movement is defective, resulting in loss of the capacity to imitate. Both forms may exist in the same patient as commands of varying complexity are presented. The anatomical implication of ideomotor apraxia is disconnection of the preserved parietal cortex from that of the frontal lobe.

Motor Apraxia

Limb-kinetic, kinetic, or motor apraxia refers to the inability to translate commands that the patient understands into purposive acts. The same acts may, however, be made reflexly, involuntarily, inadvertently, or in another context. Motor apraxia is often associated with disorders of spoken language. It usually involves both sides of the body. While gross focal lesions of the left frontal lobe result in severe bilateral motor apraxia, a focal lesion is not necessary, and decompensation of motor function with apraxia may accompany such diffuse bifrontal disorders as general paresis. Motor apraxia is easily detected by asking the patient to perform such common tasks as waving or saluting or to perform more complex acts such as combing his hair with and without utensil. The concept is clearly understood, and the patient may be able to describe what he has been asked to do. He recognizes his errors though he is unable to correct them. He can imitate, but compulsive imitation is absent. Many demented patients are able to perform stereotyped and familiar tasks with implements, though not able to act them out without utensils. Less familiar or more complex tasks may be beyond their competence. As it becomes more pervasive, motor apraxia interferes with occupational activities and later with feeding, dressing, and self-care.

Ideational, ideomotor, and motor elements of varying degree are often found together in dementia. As the dementia intensifies they become even more difficult to separate, though at all times some difficulty in recalling how to carry out an act, translating it into action, or making purposive movement upon command remains evident. Steadily and progressively the range of behavior becomes restricted and increasingly concrete. The patient has become unable to use his limbs in any conceptualized way for transactional behavior, and as he becomes helpless they are used for little but postural adjustment and automatic contactual responses.[15,62]

SPECIAL CONSIDERATIONS: UNILATERAL, GAIT, DRESSING, AND CONSTRUCTIONAL APRAXIA

Lesions of the anterior portion of the corpus callosum may be followed by loss of manual executive ability in the otherwise normal left hand. Current concepts of language function suggest that the left frontal lobe is important in the performance of skilled acts, particularly of the hand, lips, tongue, and face. If the left hand alone is to be used for writing, gesticulation, or other purposive acts, then the left frontal lobe must have access to the right motor regions. When this is lost, as in a rostral callosal or paracallosal lesion, the left limbs cannot be used for this purpose though they are otherwise normal.[30,31]

Gait apraxia, sometimes called *marche à petits pas,* *"slipping clutch" syndrome,* or *frontal lobe gait,* is a special disorder related to motor apraxia but not necessarily concomitant with it.[44] Such patients are unable to pretend that they are walking or make appropriate movements while lying, sitting, or standing. When actually walking they start with a short shuffling pace, often walking in place (the slipping clutch) or falling backward. Gait, once initiated, proceeds on a normal base but with a tendency to body and limb flexion. Reciprocal leg movements are impaired, and the patient has as much difficulty arresting or altering the rate or direction of movement as he does starting. Loss of reciprocal leg movement further impedes getting into or rising from bed for the legs are moved as though tied together. Walking becomes abnormally responsive to visual influences. Movement in the visual field may cause the patient to stop or tumble backward, and the intrusion of such common irregularities of surface as lines on a floor may arrest gait, causing the pace to shorten or the patient to walk in place. As the process worsens, progressive shortening of the length of the pace and fixed flexion of the limbs supervene. Patients ultimately become unable to walk as their limbs become fixed in flexion. Progressive incontinence of bowel and bladder may accompany the more severe gait disorder.[62]

Loss of mental power does not always parallel the gait change, and many individuals retain a level of mental competence that, though reduced, is better than the impairment of walking might suggest. A change in muscle tone that may be confused with rigidity (as in paralysis agitans) invariably appears as the gait becomes "apractic." This is variously called *paratonic rigidity, gegenhalten,* or *countermovement.* Excessive reactions are elicited upon stroking, scratching, or pressing on the sole of the foot, characterized by sustained plantar flexion of the foot and toes and inversion of the ankles (tonic foot responses) (see Chapter 2).

The upper limbs may be relatively uninvolved in cases in which gait apraxia is predominant. Conversely, the arms and hands may be involved out of proportion to the legs and feet as mechanisms related to the lateral frontal region become defective. Apraxia is bilateral (except with the rare paracallosal lesion mentioned above) and is usually associated with gross cognitive defects. Immobility and apparently contented adaptation to a fixed position are important clinical features of most apractic patients. Instinctive or reflex grasp reflexes are usually found, with compulsive palpation and manipulation frequently present.[17,50] Sequential, visually driven, or conceptualized movements of the arm and hand are diminished while contactual automatisms are released. The hand projects little into space and correspondingly remains in contact with the body surface, the other hand, or a haphazardly encountered object such as the arm of a chair or a fold of bed clothing. Highly stereotyped, compulsively repeated movements, such as rapidly slapping the thigh or touching objects, are common.

The lips, face, and tongue may become apractic.[22,30] Executive language function is usually disordered simultaneously, but the latter may occur without the former. That oral facial apraxia exists without aphasia is questionable. Except when a gross lesion of the left hemisphere is present, the usual implication of facial apraxia is that the most lateral frontal lobes have been affected bilaterally. Such patients are unable to whistle, smile, blink, scowl, protrude or retract their tongues on command, though similar movements may be made involuntarily. Some patients become apractic for eating and swallowing and must be fed by gavage. Released oral automatisms on contactual and visual stimulation usually accompany such facial apraxia. They appear to have the same significance in the face as palmar grasping or the tonic foot response. They are elicited by gentle finger stroke along the nasolabial fold and the corner of the mouth, which results in retraction of the corner of the mouth and pursing the lips toward the stimulus with adversion of the head and eyes.[19]

Eye movements may reduce in number, rate per minute, and range with bifrontal disorders. Staring and ocular immobility lead to a fixed facies that may be confused with parkinsonism. Eye movements become less discrete, encompassing a rather narrow range before the head begins to turn. Patterns of ocular search have similarly been shown to be of small excursion and limited to a few movements at a prolonged latency and rate. Ocular motility thus resembles all other patterns of movement in such patients, tending to be stereotyped, dependent upon highly specific stimuli, and vulnerable to extinction by interruption.[42,55] This generalization may be useful as a guide to the clinical interpretation of nonparalytic impairment of motility in dementing disease.

The quality and competence of movements become defective as their latency, rate, and range become affected. Such incompetence becomes increasingly evident as attempted activities are less habitual, more protracted (hence more vulnerable to distraction), and increasingly dependent on conceptualization, planning, and memory. Highly customary movements and those subject to regulation by continuing visual or sensory control are least affected. The apractic state interferes chiefly with mentally projected and temporally extensive movements. Planning thus becomes defective, and stereotyped thoughts and acts superimposed upon immobility. Mildly apractic patients may realize their deficiencies and become depressed reactively.

Constructional and *dressing apraxia* are confusing terms as they refer to highly specific consequences of perceptual and agnosic disorders. They are usually encountered together and associated with focal lesions of either parietotemporal region, though more frequently with the non-dominant side. Constructional apraxia, occurring in either focal or diffuse cerebral disease, is easily demonstrated and is the basis of many psychological tests of "visuomotor incoordination." It may be demonstrated by requiring the patient to assemble sticks according to a pattern shown by the examiner or to copy a design such as two unequal, asymmetrical pentagons each of which intersects the other on two successive sides. The behavioral consequence of constructional apraxia is incompetence to arrange objects in space relative to one another owing to inability to discern their spatial relationships. Side-to-side confusion, finger agnosia, and impaired calculation are usually found at the same time. When the constructional disorder follows a gross parietal lesion, the side of the figure opposite the cerebral lesion is omitted on attempted copying but the angular relationships are retained. When the process is diffuse or the patient aphasic, the whole figure becomes altered in size and shape, tending in general to simplification. A pentagon may thus be reproduced as a square.

Confusion for body side and part may also be associated with disordered dressing (dressing apraxia). Grooming, shaving, bathing, and combing the hair are neglected or incomplete. Clothing, including spectacles, false teeth, and bed covers, is put on incorrectly. Like constructional apraxia, disordered dressing may result from a gross temporoparietal lesion, more often on the non-dominant side. In that case the disorder of dressing is more defective on the side opposite the cerebral lesion. Patients fail to clothe or cover that side of the body and neglect to shave that side of the face. Since dressing and constructional apraxia are accompanied by defective awareness, patients do not complain about them or understand the complaints of others, frequently placing the blame for their failures elsewhere.[5,21,59]

APHASIC MANIFESTATIONS

Language content and competency of the demented patient may be affected independently of memory, cognition, and motility, though usually each is altered to some degree and each deficiency interacts with the others. The content of the demented patient's language may reflect abnormalities of thinking, such as concreteness, which are part of the general dementing disorder.[7,35] The quality of grammatical construction and syntax may deteriorate as simple sentences convey little information or thought. Relatively specific attributes of aphasic disorders, such as impaired fluency or paraphasic speech, may further diminish the use of language. The former two conditions usually accompany dementing states secondary to diffuse disease; the latter, focal or more severe disease of the left cerebrum.

Language incompetence develops at a rate and to a degree corresponding to other changes in function that occur in the underlying dementing condition. The patient speaks less often and says less when he does so. Utterances become increasingly stereotyped, perseverative, and concrete; abstractions and symbolization disappear from language. The vocal volume may be reduced and the tone high pitched, curiously querulous, or cracking. Auditory comprehension suffers as concrete language is better understood than abstract. When auditory incomprehension is prominent, patients may talk excessively, rambling on in irrelevant and disorganized sentences or sentence fragments, often responding to every environmental sound. Reading comprehension becomes less efficient, and writing becomes cramped and poorly formed, the content contaminated by grammatical, spelling, syntactical, and perseverative errors. These deficiencies are encountered frequently in diffuse conditions such as Alzheimer's disease, senile dementia, and general paresis.

The progressive concretization of language may be accompanied by compulsive reiteration of simple phrases (often prayer fragments or obscenities) that are either meaningless or out of context. Spoken language thus becomes a litany of expostulations or old sayings devoid of conceptual or ideational content. Facial apraxia and immobility are often present. Facial expression no longer indicates the content and intent of speech and may be further altered by developing tremors of the lips and tongue. Compulsive chewing, lip smacking, or protrusion and retraction of the tongue may be evoked or intensified by attempting to talk. Pseudobulbar palsy with spastic dysarthria and altered respiratory rhythm further alter articulation. The resulting abnormality of language content, competence, and quality, reflecting the extent of the dementia, isolates the patient from normal, uncomprehending people. Patients may then respond "catastrophically" with agitation or withdrawal.

Aphasic changes in dementia differ in clinical appearance from those consequent upon gross focal disease. The demented patient ordinarily acquires his language disorder within the context of widespread brain disease. Multiple language attributes are affected simultaneously, and the resulting aphasic deficit though mild may be subtle and complex. Aphasic features evolve gradually in degenerative diseases and tend to reflect the chief locus of pathology. In the case of patients whose dementia begins with visual agnosia, like the man described earlier, reading comprehension may be impaired out of proportion to executive speech or auditory comprehension. The implication of such a lexical disorder is affection of mechanisms dependent upon the dominant parietal lobe.[34] Writing usually deteriorates at the same time that reading is becoming abnormal. Calligraphy becomes irregular; lines are not followed; words are misspelled; and syntactical errors interfere with content. The lexical disability interferes with recognition of the mistakes as the patient cannot read his own writing.

APHASIC MANIFESTATIONS OF FOCAL DISEASE

The capacity to understand spoken language (and such associated functions as the ability to recall names on description or on visual, auditory, or tactile presentation, and the ability to write to dictation) may become defective as disease affects mechanisms related to the dominant temporal and lateral parietal regions.[34] Jargon fragments may be heard, and phrases or cognate words substituted for forgotten names, nouns, or verbs (paraphasia). These elements may be mixed with auditory hallucinations and paranoid behavior.

Echopraxia, echolalia, and perseveration emerge as comprehension becomes more defective. The ability to repeat spoken language may be spared. As incomprehension worsens, fragments of language, newly formed words, and isolated syllables dominate spoken speech, which is thus reduced to an unintelligible jargon. Auditory comprehension occasionally becomes so impaired that the patient is word deaf and mute for practical purposes. Progressive dementing illnesses that begin in the posterior hemisphere may thus result in an aphasic state marked by lexical, auditory, nominal, amnestic, and syntactical elements. When widespread disease involves the nondominant hemisphere as well, disorders of visual, somesthetic, and auditory perception accompany the language disorder. The aphasic features themselves are not unique, but the total context of the disorder is. In contrast, when similar aphasia develops in patients with focal disease, it remains isolated and free of the general disintegration that characterizes bilateral diffuse disease.

Disorders that involve the frontal lobes, such as general paresis, Pick's disease, and some cases of senile dementia, may disturb fluency, articulation, writing, gesture, and pantomime.[4,34,35] Executive speech, writing, and gesture are usually greatly impaired when focal disease is gross, but in most dementing conditions the local pathology is not intense though widespread. Spontaneous language is reduced. Speech occurs less often and somewhat more slowly; the sentences tend toward simple declarations. Verbal stereotypy becomes pronounced with the same phrases being repeated over and over. Fewer words are used in active speech, though vocabulary remains broad. Articulation is altered with individual syllables being mispronounced; the patient may stammer. Handwriting reflects the changes in speech as it becomes cramped and ill formed. Words are often left incomplete as only the initial letters are written. Frequently the patient is so apractic for writing (apractic agraphia) that he cannot manipulate a pencil or simply scribbles repetitively. This is contrasted with relative preservation of the formation of letters in the patient with a lexical disorder. Pantomime and gesture may become distorted and incomprehensible, the change reflecting the underlying disorder of spoken and written language. Gesture tends to disappear in frontally based disorders.

Executive language is not totally lost without other neurological deficit in dementia. Mutism, apractic agraphia, and loss of pantomime without any other language disorder are theoretical constructs that may be of heuristic value but are quite divorced from reality. In conditions like Pick's disease, impaired executive language soon becomes associated with loss of memory for words (amnestic or nominal aphasia) [43] and paraphasia appears. Paraphasia and syntactical disorganization increase with loss of fluency.[40] The tendency thus is toward impaired language expression and auditory incomprehension. The apparently specific disorder of executive speech may only reflect a bias in the distribution of the pathology, the proportion of symptoms present at any time, or the completeness of examination.[41]

Impaired fluency and articulation, apractic agraphia, and loss of pantomime usually coexist with other features of bifrontal disease—reduced activity, impoverished or stereotyped movements, apparent depression of mood, and motor apraxia—all of which may mask the attendant aphasic features. The agitated depression that accompanies aphasia in focal cerebral disease is usually absent as the general effect of the illness on intellect diminishes the patient's understanding of what is happening to him. The aphasic aspect of dementing disease is usually associated with equally severe disorders of cognitive function, while focal disease usually spares intellectual function.

Pseudobulbar palsy (spastic dysphagia and dysarthria, emotional lability with forced laughing and crying, and periodic respiration and pulse) may be present along with aphasic features. Pseudobulbar manifestations usually mean affection of subcortical structures and do not ordinarily occur until neuronal disease is severe. Apractic dysphagia, aphasic dysarthria, and emotional impoverishment or inappropriateness, however, are more characteristic of nerve-cell disease. Pronounced pseudobulbar states are usually, but not necessarily, accompanied by some degree of dementia. A consistent feature of pseudobulbar palsy is the fixed facial attitude in which the forehead is wrinkled, the brows elevated, the palpebral fissures widened, and the corners of the mouth retracted. Dystonic flexion of the legs and reduced use of the arms without apraxia may cause confusion with paralysis agitans.[16] Fixed pseudobulbar manifestations are most often encountered in hypertensive and diabetic patients who have many small bilaterally placed lesions in the cerebral white matter, corticobulbar tracts, caudate nucleus, putamen, and globus pallidus. Similarly placed lesions may occur after hypoxia and in Wilson's disease and Huntington's chorea. The faciopharyngeal and appendicular symptom clusters are usually commingled. The former are attributed to the corticobulbar lesions and the latter to those in the caudate nucleus and putamen.

A new focal cerebral lesion in a previously demented patient may be attended by widespread functional decompensation, in contrast to the effect of the same lesion in a normal or nearly normal person. A mildly apractic patient may, for example, develop an attitude of upper limb flexion and be transiently unable to use his arms for purposive acts following infarction of an occipital lobe. The consequences on language function might be mutism, auditory incomprehension, inattentiveness to spoken language, or agitated delirium.[39] Such decompensation occurs frequently in patients with cerebral vascular disease. While patients who have undergone catastrophic decompensation may improve, others decline progressively, especially when the underlying mechanism is hypoxia. Continuing deterioration in diffuse disorders maintains a state of chronic decompensation.

SUMMARY

Symptoms of amnesia, agnosia, apraxia, and aphasia occur alone and in combination in dementia. They indicate functional impairment of appropriately localized parts of the brain, but the dementia cannot be explained by their simple arithmetic sum as other elements also contribute to the deterioration of intellect. When dementia results from diffuse brain disease, and personality and behavior have undergone extensive alteration, memory, cognition, motility, and language are all defective. Each deficit may vary somewhat in its relative intensity, and each is embedded in a complex matrix. Amnesia, agnosia, apraxia, and aphasia develop to a degree and evolve at a rate that reflects the nature and progress of the underlying illness. Memory, language, cognition, and motility are usually mildly or at most moderately impaired until diffuse brain disease has become severely destructive.

Bilateral symmetrical lobar involvement may affect memory, cognition, motility, or language in a relatively individual manner, sparing the other disproportionately, but there is invariably some more general alteration of the totality of personality, intellect, and behavior. Gross lateralized deficits are absent in both diffuse and bilobar conditions.

Dementia may also complicate extensive focal disease of either cerebral hemisphere. In this instance the total intellectual function of the patient may be somewhat reduced, but aphasia, agnosia, or apraxia may occur alone and exceed in severity that encountered in any but the most severe diffuse condition. Signs attributable to extensive localized brain disease such as hemiplegia, hemianesthesia, or hemianopia are overwhelming. Despite gross deficits in one or more of the functions considered in this chapter, others may escape nearly completely.

For practical clinical purposes dementia cannot safely be attributed to a single focal cerebral lesion unless signs of gross hemispheric decompensation are present. Dementia cannot safely be attributed to diffuse or widespread disease unless multiple deficits are demonstrated. Focal lesions of the brain that cause dementia have usually compromised the affected hemisphere widely, and reports of curing dementia by treating local conditions excepting subdural hematoma should be regarded critically. Conversely, diffuse involvement of the brain does not necessarily indicate an untreatable or irremediable disorder.

REFERENCES

1. ADLER, A.: *Disintegration and restoration of optic recognition in visual agnosia.* Arch. Neurol. Psychiat. 51:243, 1944.

2. ADLER, A.: *Course and outcome of visual agnosia.* J. Nerv. Ment. Dis. 111: 41, 1950.

3. ALAJOUANINE, T., AND LHERMITTE, F.: Some problems concerning the agnosias, apraxia, and aphasia, in Halpern, L. (ed.): *Problems of Dynamic Neurology.* Hebrew Univ., Hadassah Medical School, Jerusalem, Israel, 1963, pp. 201-216.

4. ALLISON, R. S.: *The Senile Brain.* Arnold, London, 1962.

5. ARRIGONI, G., AND DE RENZI, E.: *Constructional apraxia and hemispheric locus of lesion.* Cortex 1:170, 1964.

6. BAY, E.: *Disturbances of visual perception and their examination.* Brain 76:515, 1953.

7. BAY, E.: Aphasia and conceptual thinking, in Halpern, L. (ed.): *Problems of Dynamic Neurology.* Hebrew Univ., Hadassah Medical School, Jerusalem, Israel, 1963, pp. 88-100.

8. BAY, E.: *Problems, possibilities, and limitations of localization of psychic symptoms in the brain.* Cortex 1:91, 1964.

9. BENDER, M. B.: *Disorders in Perception.* Charles C Thomas, Publisher, Springfield, Ill., 1952.

10. BENDER, M. B.: Disorders in visual perception, in Halpern, L. (ed.): *Problems of Dynamic Neurology.* Hebrew Univ., Hadassah Medical School, Jerusalem, Israel, 1963, pp. 319-375.

11. BICKFORD, R. G., MULDER, D. W., DODGE, H. W., JR., SVIEN, H. J., AND ROME, H. P.: Changes in memory function produced by electrical stimulation of the temporal lobe in man, in *The Brain and Human Behavior.* Proc. Assoc. Res. Nerv. Ment. Dis. The Williams & Wilkins Co., Baltimore, Vol. XXXVI, 1958, pp. 227-243.

12. BRAIN, W. R.: Disorders of memory, in Brain, W. R., and Wilkinson, M. (eds.): *Recent Advances in Neurology and Neuropsychiatry,* ed. 8, Churchill, London, 1969, pp. 1-12.

13. CRITCHLEY, M.: *The Parietal Lobes.* Arnold, London, 1953.

14. DEJONG, R. N., ITABASHI, H. H., AND OLSON, J. R.: *"Pure" memory loss with hippocampal lesions: A case report.* Trans. Amer. Neurol. Assn. 93:31, 1968.

15. DENNY-BROWN, D.: *Disintegration of motor function resulting from cerebral lesions.* J. Nerv. Ment. Dis. 112:1, 1950.

16. DENNY-BROWN, D.: Focal lesions of the basal ganglia, in *The Basal Ganglia and Their Relation to Disorders of Movement*. Oxford University Press, London, 1962, Chap. 3, pp. 53-70.

17. DENNY-BROWN, D.: The frontal lobes and their functions, in Feiling, A. (ed.) : *Modern Trends in Neurology*. Hoeber, New York, 1951, pp. 13-89.

18. DENNY-BROWN, D.: *The nature of apraxia*. J. Nerv. Ment. Dis. 126:9, 1958.

19. DENNY-BROWN, D.: *Positive and negative aspects of cerebral cortical function*. N. Carolina Med. J. 17:295, 1956.

20. DENNY-BROWN, D., AND CHAMBERS, R. A.: The parietal lobe and behavior, in *The Brain and Human Behavior*. Proc. Assoc. Res. Nerv. Ment. Dis. The Williams & Wilkins Co., Baltimore, Vol. XXXVI, 1958, pp. 35-117.

21. DENNY-BROWN, D., MEYER, J. S., AND HORENSTEIN, S.: *The significance of perceptual rivalry resulting from parietal lesion*. Brain 75:433, 1952.

22. DE RENZI, E., PIECZARO, A., AND VIGNOLO, L. A.: *Oral apraxia and aphasia*. Cortex 2:50, 1966.

23. DRACHMAN, D. A., AND ARBIT, J.: *Memory and the hippocampal complex, II*. Arch. Neurol. 15:52, 1966.

24. DRACHMAN, D. A., AND OMMAYA, A. K.: *Memory and the hippocampal complex*. Arch. Neurol. 10:411, 1964.

25. EBBINGHAUS, H.: *Memory: A Contribution to Experimental Psychology*. 1885. Republished by Dover Publications, New York, 1964.

26. ETTLINGER, G. G. (ed.) : *Functions of the Corpus Callosum*. Little, Brown and Company, Boston, 1965.

27. FISHER, C. M., AND ADAMS, R. D.: *Transient global amnesia*. Acta Neurol. Scand. (Suppl. 9) 40:1, 1964.

28. GESCHWIND, N.: The anatomy of acquired disorders of reading, in Money, J.: *Reading Disability*. The Johns Hopkins Press, Baltimore, 1962, pp. 115-130.

29. GESCHWIND, N.: *Disconnexion syndromes in animals and man. Part I*. Brain 88:237, 1965.

30. GESCHWIND, N.: *Disconnexion syndromes in animals and man. Part II*. Brain 88:585, 1965.

31. GESCHWIND, N., AND KAPLAN, E.: *A human cerebral disconnection syndrome*. Neurology 12:675, 1962.

32. GILMAN, S.: *Cerebral disorders after open heart operations*. New Eng. J. Med. 272:489, 1965.

33. HÉCAEN, H., DE AJURIAGUERRA, J., AND ANGELERGUES, R.: Apraxia and its various aspects, in Halpern, L. (ed.) : *Problems of Dynamic Neurology*. Hebrew Univ., Hadassah Medical School, Jerusalem, Israel, 1963, pp. 217-230.

34. HÉCAEN, H., AND ANGELERGUES, R.: Localization of symptoms in aphasia, in deReuck, A. V. S., and O'Connor, M. (eds.) : *Disorders of Language*. Little, Brown and Company, Boston, 1964, pp. 223-260.

35. Hécaen, H., and Angelergues, R.: *Pathologie du language l'aphasie.* Larousse, Paris, 1965, pp. 141-157, 177-182.

36. Horenstein, S., and Casey, T. R.: *Paropsis associated with hemianopia.* Trans. Amer. Neurol. Assn. 89:204, 1964.

37. Horenstein, S., and Casey, T. R.: *Perceptual defects in both visual fields in attention hemianopia.* Trans. Amer. Neurol. Assn. 88:60, 1963.

38. Horenstein, S., Casey, T. R., and Gardner, J. H.: *Disturbance of gaze and fixation in hemianopic patients in disturbance of the occipital lobe.* Proc. 8th Int. Cong. of Neurology, Vienna, Vol. III, 1965, pp. 253-257.

39. Horenstein, S., Chamberlin, W., and Conomy, J.: *Infarction of the fusiform and calcarine regions: Agitated delirium and hemianopia.* Trans. Amer. Neurol. Assn. 92:85, 1967.

40. Irigaray, L.: *Approche psycho-linguistique du langage des dements.* Neuropsychologia 5:25, 1967.

41. Luria, A. R.: Factors and forms of aphasia, in deReuck, A. V. S., and O'Connor, M. (eds.) : *Disorders of Language.* Little, Brown and Company, Boston, 1964, pp. 143-167.

42. Luria, A. R., Karpon, B. A., and Yarbus, A. L.: *Disturbances of active visual perception with lesions of the frontal lobes.* Cortex 2:202, 1966.

43. Luria, A. R., Sokolov, E. M., and Klimkowski, M.: *Towards a neurodynamic analysis of memory disturbances with lesions of the left temporal lobe.* Neuropsychologia 5:1, 1967.

44. Meyer, J. S., and Barron, D. W.: *Apraxia of gait: A clinico-physiological study.* Brain 83:261, 1960.

45. Milner, B.: Psychological defects produced by temporal lobe excision, in *The Brain and Human Behavior.* Proc. Assoc. Res. Nerv. Ment. Dis. The Williams & Wilkins Company, Baltimore, Vol. XXXVI, 1958, pp. 244-257.

46. Mitchell, J.: *Speech and language impairment in the older patient.* Geriatrics 13:467, 1958.

47. Reinhold, M.: *A case of auditory agnosia.* Brain 73:203, 1950.

48. Russell, W. R.: *Brain, Memory, Learning.* Oxford University Press, London, 1959.

49. Russell, W. R., and Nathan, P.: *Traumatic amnesia.* Brain 69:280, 1946.

50. Seyffarth, H., and Denny-Brown, D.: *The grasp reflex and the instinctive grasp reaction.* Brain 71:109, 1948.

51. Sperry, R. W.: *Hemisphere deconnection and unity in conscious awareness.* Amer. Psychol. 23:723, 1968.

52. Stengel, E.: Speech disorder and mental disorders, in deReuck, A. V. S., and O'Connor, M. (eds.) : *Disorders of Language.* Little, Brown and Company, Boston, 1964, pp. 285-298.

53. Sweet, W. H., Talland, G. A., and Ervin, F. R.: *Loss of recent memory following section of the fornix.* Trans. Amer. Neurol. Assn. 84:76, 1959.

54. Tyler, H. R.: *Abnormalities of perception with defective eye movements (Balint's syndrome).* Cortex 4:154, 1968.

55. TYLER, H. R.: Disorders of visual scanning with frontal lobe lesions, in Locke, S. (ed.) : *Modern Neurology. Papers in Tribute to Derek Denny-Brown.* Little, Brown and Company, Boston, 1969, pp. 381-394.

56. VICTOR, M.: Observations on the amnestic syndrome in man and its anatomical basis, in Brazier, M. A. B. (ed.) : *Brain Function. II. RNA and Brain Function, Memory, and Learning.* University of California Press, Berkeley, Calif., 1964, pp. 311-337.

57. WEINSTEIN, E. A., AND KAHN, R. L.: *Denial of Illness: Symbolic and Physiological Aspects.* Charles C Thomas, Publisher, Springfield, Ill., 1955.

58. WEINSTEIN, E. A., AND KAHN, R. L.: *Non-aphasic misnaming (paraphasia) in organic brain disease.* Arch. Neurol. Psychiat. 67:72, 1952.

59. WEINSTEIN, E. A., AND KAHN, R. L.: *Syndrome of anosognosia.* Arch. Neurol. Psychiat. 64:772, 1950.

60. WHITTY, C. W. M.: The neurological basis of memory, in Williams, D. (ed.) : *Modern Trends in Neurology 3.* Butterworth, London, 1962, pp. 314-335.

61. WHITTY, C. W. M., AND LISHMAN, W. A.: Amnesia in cerebral disease, in Whitty, C. W. M., and Zangwill, O. L. (eds.) : *Amnesia.* Butterworth, London, 1966, pp. 36-76.

62. YAKOVLEV, P. I.: *Paralysis in flexion of cerebral origin.* J. Neuropath. Exp. Neurol. 13:267, 1954.

Chapter 4

The Clinical Use of Psychological Testing in Dementia

Simon Horenstein, M.D.

Psychological testing may be profitable in the clinical evaluation, treatment, and rehabilitation of the demented patient. Its usefulness depends largely on what questions are formulated by the physician and the availability of a psychologist skilled and experienced in the study of organic brain disease. Psychological testing appears especially helpful in defining original or native intelligence and its deterioration, and in segregating the varieties and degrees of cognitive defect, memory loss, and language impairment. Testing appears less precise in identifying disorders of judgment and conation. Personality mechanisms, interests, and aptitudes may also be explored and the results used in planning management or rehabilitation. Such testing is largely limited to patients who retain some capacity to comprehend and comply with the situational demands of the tests. Fatigue, experience, and such emotional states as depression, hunger, and fear may affect test performance, and evaluation may require several sessions. Highly individualized and descriptive interpretations are often necessary in defining conative functions, though memory, perceptual motor coordination, and language may be described relatively efficiently and quantitatively. This disparity between conative and perceptual or cognitive functions has been reduced in modern test batteries.

It is still difficult to define that behavior which reflects loss of brain function and to distinguish it from characterological or psychological disturbances in patients with frontal or temporal brain lesions. However vexing this problem, psychological methods can contribute to the study of most demented patients. The physician should not, however, expect testing to "make the diagnosis" of dementia or to identify the specific disease causing the intellectual change. Recognition of dementia as well as the specific clinical or pathological diagnosis should be inferred from the sum of history, physical examination, and pertinent diagnostic procedures including psychological testing.

Psychological testing may attain one or more of five goals: (1) quantification of a presumed deficit in intelligence, whether developmental or acquired; (2) definition and differentiation of cognitive, agnosic, aphasic, and amnestic elements; (3) documentation of the resolution, dissolution, or progression of the behavioral consequences of an illness; (4) assistance in planning followup or comprehensive care of individual patients, particularly by identifying interests and aptitudes; and (5) separation of dementing symptoms from others related to premorbid personality or emotional response to illness.

INTELLIGENCE TESTS

Tests designed to measure "native intelligence" have been used to predict school performance and establish the degree of mental deficiency since the earliest instruments devised by Binet. They have consisted of a cluster of subtests designed to explore abilities judged important in academic success. They have generally been designed around scholastic information emphasizing complex skills including problem solving, symbol formulation and manipulation, vocabulary, and information. They have been designed for administration under a variety of language-dependent visual and auditory conditions. These attributes limit their validity in patients whose social, cultural, and educational backgrounds are very different from those of the essentially literate, urban population for whom the tests were designed and in whom they have proved reliable, dependable, and efficient.

Most demented patients are older and their school years long past. They have accumulated experience, control, and wisdom with maturity though speed and flexibility have become reduced. Tests designed for children are inappropriate either to evaluate their original intelligence or to identify mental deterioration. Instruments have been created to compensate for age and natural loss of mental efficiency. The Wechsler Adult Intelligence Scale (WAIS) is the most widely used of individually administered tests designed to study adult intelligence. It is successor to the Wechsler-Bellevue Intelligence Test (WBIT). Both the WBIT and WAIS permit individuals to be scored within age groups between 16 and 64 years, to compensate for the effects of aging on tested intelligence.* Within this age range, this efficient test provides a measure of both original and residual intellectual ability as well as a measure of the difference between them. Its reliability additionally permits reexamination of the patient with little fear of improvement by practice. The test has also been standardized on an older population and norms established through and beyond age 75 years.

The WAIS is divided into 11 subtests: 6 verbal (information, comprehension, arithmetic, similarities, digit span, and vocabulary) and 5 performance (digit symbol, picture completion, block design, picture arrangement, and object assembly). The subtest scores vary little from one another in normal and retarded persons. The scores earned on the subtests are summed to give verbal and performance scores that are respectively converted into verbal and performance I.Q.'s by reference to an age-specific table. The latter are combined to provide a "full-scale" I.Q.

The verbal and performance I.Q.'s are usually within a few points of one another, but in organic disorders (other than severely aphasic states) the verbal score usually exceeds the performance. Preserved functions help indicate original intelligence, and lost ones, the effect of disease. Similarities, digit span, digit symbol, and block design are tests that are vulnerable to organic disease of the brain without respect to cause. These "don't hold" items appear to be relatively independent of prior learning, and their successful completion depends on the patient's capacity to perform new associations and manipulate symbols. Information, vocabulary, picture completion, and object assembly ("hold" items) are said to be resistant to deterioration and hence regarded as useful indicators of premorbid intelligence. A "deterioration index" may be calculated from the hold and don't hold scores. This quotient is normally close

---

*For discussion of this topic, see Chapter 9.

to 1, and losses of 15 to 20 per cent are regarded as significant. This figure is viewed in relation to subtest scores, especially those of comprehension and picture arrangement. Not all psychologists concur in the validity of the deterioration index, some preferring to depend upon the relationship between verbal and performance scores. The full-scale score is thought by others to be more reliable in identifying deterioration, particularly when dealing with an individual whose life accomplishments or prior test results indicate intelligence superior to that disclosed by the most recent evaluation. Low subtest scores are readily identified. Such intertest "scatter" often points to areas deserving specialized or more intensive investigation.

The estimation of "native intelligence" in the presence of illiteracy or cultural heterogeneity has been approached by tests, such as the Army Beta of World War I, that do not require highly developed scholastic skills. They are composed of subtests covering areas of information, picture completion, object arrangement, vocabulary, comprehension, judgment, and problem solving. Individually administered, such tests require no reading. The Arthur Point Scale of Performance Tests is a battery of tests involving manipulation of form, reproduction of design, and solution of mazes directed to nonreading, non-English-speaking, deaf, or language-handicapped patients. The Peabody Picture Vocabulary Test and the Raven Progressive Matrices, the latter originally a group test, are also administered to individuals. The former has the advantage of testing vocabulary without required reading. The latter requires the patient to match progressively difficult figures and designs and is said to correlate well with more comprehensive tests. Although often helpful in establishing the probabilities of native intelligence, these tests are less quantitative and more subject to variability. Individual psychometrists often become quite skilled in administering and interpreting them, and the results obtained may contribute to the separation of the demented from the culturally deprived.

Group testing of intelligence has been widely used in school systems for periodic testing of intelligence and predicting academic performance, usually two or three times at 3- to 4-year intervals during a child's school career. The Army General Classification Test has been used to establish levels of intellectual competence in military personnel for nearly 30 years. Group tests are not ordinarily applied to the study of demented individuals, but test results obtained from school or military records may facilitate interpretation of the results of testing after the onset of disease.

In conditions that begin with defective visual recognition, such as may occur in Alzheimer's disease, gross abnormalities may be anticipated in those WAIS subtests that depend upon capacity to arrange components into an object, complete or arrange pictures into logical sequences, substitute symbols for digits, or arrange blocks after a pictured design. While the full-scale I.Q. is reduced, selective reduction is found in specific performance items. Conversely, in Korsakoff's dementia, the storage, integration, recall, and reproduction of memory are affected out of proportion to other mental attributes. Tests of digit span (the number of random digits that the patient can repeat forward and backward) and digit symbol (a test that requires the patient to substitute a geometric symbol for an arabic numeral) depend largely upon retention and recall; hence, in Korsakoff's dementia they may be markedly impaired relative to fairly well preserved vocabulary, information, and the capacity to recognize missing parts (picture completion), arrange pictures logically (picture arrangement), or reproduce designs by arranging blocks (block design). Thus, the use of techniques originally designed to estimate "native intelligence" may lead to recognition and quantification of the specific impairments that characterize the clinical disorder.

Knowledge of the nature and magnitude of specific defects also helps in planning therapeutic or rehabilitative programs and in counseling the patient and his family. As suggested in the preceding examples of Alzheimer's disease and Korsakoff's dementia, delineation of "specific" mental deficits ordinarily proceeds from observed inequality or "scatter" among WAIS subtest scores.

In organic brain disease, vocabulary, information, and comprehension scores are generally higher than the average of the subtest scores. Comprehension may, however, be severely affected by extensive frontal and callosal pathology and vocabulary altered when patients suffer any degree of aphasia. Digit span, digit symbol, block design, and object assembly—test items that depend on concentration, memory, and new associations—are most seriously affected. Depression of the former two reflects disordered memory and of the latter, disturbed visual perceptual function. Other test items are usually less severely affected in mild to moderate conditions, and the verbal is generally superior to the performance score. Deviation between verbal and performance scores and marked interest variation suggest an acquired disorder. The hold score usually exceeds the don't hold in these conditions. Thus, visuomotor function, memory, and the capacity to learn, organize, and synthesize become impaired pari passu with advancing mental inflexibility. In mental retardation one is more likely to see rather uniform depression of subtests except for object assembly which is higher and arithmetic which is usually lower by far. Additional factors used to complete the psychological evaluation may include reference to results of prior group testing and comparison of test results with those obtained in age-matched controls (a factor built into the WAIS) and with scores estimated or anticipated from the patient's educational attainments and occupational history. Identification of the cause and anatomical locus of the underlying condition is not the chief goal of testing, however reliably the psychological features of organic brain disease may be detected. Neurological signs, after all, are rarely disease specific, and higher cerebral functions rarely depend upon discrete cerebral foci.

COGNITION

Specific cognitive deficits may be studied further by using tests specifically designed for the purpose. Among those commonly employed for quantitative and qualitative study of defects in cognition, abstraction, or reasoning is the five-part group known as the Goldstein-Scheerer Test of Abstract and Concrete Thinking. One of these, the Goldstein-Scheerer Cube Test, requires the patient to assemble varicolored blocks in patterns resembling those shown him on cards. The difficulty is graded and ultimately presents reduced figures that provide no clues as to the number of blocks needed. The Weigle-Goldstein-Scheerer Color-Form Sorting Test is solved first by sorting either by shape or color a set of four squares, circles, and triangles of different colors. Having sorted them one way, the patient is then asked to rearrange them according to another principle, testing thereby his capacity to shift from one solution to another. The Goldstein-Scheerer Stick Test explores the ability to reproduce simple figures by arranging sticks of various lengths. A box of wool skeins is sorted according to color in the Gelb-Goldstein Color Sorting Test. The Goldstein-Scheerer Object Sorting Test presents an assortment of common objects—such as plates, spoons, knives, and screwdrivers—that may be sorted variously by name, nature, or class. This test battery attempts to provide a measure of conceptualization. It has been criticized on the basis of difficulty in validation and absence of data on reliability, the influence of age, the influence of intelligence, and other factors.

The Rorschach Inkblot, Draw a Person, Bender-Gestalt, and formboard tests are also used to evaluate visual- and somesthetic-dependent cognitive and motor functions. The Rorschach and Bender-Gestalt Tests are more widely used than others in this category and are regarded as sensitive indicators. In the former the patient is asked to describe what he sees in black and white and multicolored inkblots and in the latter to copy a series of geometric patterns. The tests are said to define visuomotor and somatomotor association patterns by exploring the ability to abstract, synthesize, shift from one thought pattern to another, discriminate color and form, and organize material. Personality characteristics are also disclosed by the Rorschach and Bender. Particular attention is paid on the Rorschach to responses that organize whole cards and express movements. The meaning created is said to express personality traits and psychological mechanisms of the patient. The rotation or distortion of figures, commission and correction of errors, and maturity of construction on the Bender are similarly used. These tests frequently help to identify overall reduction in intellectual efficiency and provide information about the "texture" of a disorder. Their contribution in assessing residual ability and potential avenues of learning following brain damage is important in planning education and rehabilitation.

Memory may be tested in adults by means of the Wechsler Memory Scale, a brief, easily administered test composed of seven parts emphasizing logical memory, digit span forward and backward, and the ability to count backward quickly and accurately. Numerous tests have been devised to define aphasic defects such as Schuell's Minnesota Test for Differential Diagnosis of Aphasia and the Halstead-Wepman Aphasia Screening Test.

PERSONALITY AND PROJECTIVE TESTS

Personality and projective tests are designed to explore the feelings, personality patterns, and psychological devices peculiar to the individual patient. The projective tests allow him a great deal of latitude since the patient is asked to create responses to unstructured, meaningless, or ambiguous stimuli. His creations are believed to disclose personality traits and trends, defense mechanisms, psychological conflicts, and intellectual efficiency. These procedures may disclose some of the preexisting personality patterns of demented patients as well as the psychological mechanisms used at the time of the examination. Projection, denial, depression, displacement, somatic and referential delusions, hostility, and other mechanisms are commonly expressed by mildly affected patients. As the dementing process worsens and mental activity shrivels, patients become less and less able to project their psychological mechanisms, and projective testing becomes more literal and stereotyped. The Rorschach, Bender-Gestalt, and Draw a Person Tests have been found useful in identifying personality mechanisms and their alteration; they may be used chiefly for this purpose in persons who are not demented. Systems of interpretation of these and other projective tests have been highly criticized owing to their subjective nature and difficulty in reproduction. Aging and some of the reactive changes listed previously influence the tests. The Thematic Apperception Test (TAT), the Picture Arrangement Test, various sentence completion tests, and self-administered personality inventories such as the Minnesota Multiphasic Personality Inventory are infrequently applied to demented patients. Many psychologists also use a "clinical interview" in which the patient's dress, facial expression, gesture, language function, and thought content are noted. For many it serves as a guide in test selection.

TESTING APTITUDE AND SPECIAL INTERESTS

Special interest and aptitude tests are occasionally useful in management of the demented patient who has reached a stationary or stable level, as might be found after recovery from trauma, hypoxia, hypoglycemia, or a subarachnoid hemorrhage. These tests aim to discover specific interests or abilities, knowledge of which is valuable in guiding patients toward vocational retraining and social rehabilitation. The variety of preference scales includes the Strong, Kuder, Minnesota Multiple Abilities Test, and the General Aptitude Test Battery of the U.S. Employment Service. The first two are widely used in defining preference for broad occupational areas and appear to be rather reliable. Aptitude tests for specific skills are available for exploration in areas of preference. Many of the latter are administered by various bureaus of vocational rehabilitation operated by state employment services or other rehabilitation agencies. They appear to be reliable predictors of success.

Operation of a motor vehicle is a frequent problem, and physicians are commonly called upon for advice. Various devices have been designed to evaluate fitness to operate a motor vehicle. They depend upon actual responses to simulated traffic scenes. They are often available through automobile associations, rehabilitation centers, and driver-education programs. These tests rate such important factors as reaction time, fatigability, judgment, and impulse control.

EXAMPLES OF THE APPLICATION OF TESTING

The value of the information derived from testing largely depends on the clarity with which the problem is presented to the psychologist. The first question in any case of presumed dementia is whether intellectual deterioration has occurred and, if so, what is its nature. It is usually answered by an intelligence scale such as the WAIS, possibly expanded by additional tests such as the Bender-Gestalt and Rorschach. The latter are used to identify and quantify cognitive defects and additionally define personality mechanisms. The second question is whether mental deterioration is continuing, has achieved stability, or begun to improve. Repetition of a prior battery usually answers this question, but several weeks or months may be required between testing, especially when the illness has been toxic, traumatic, or hypoxic. The last question relates to rehabilitation. The WAIS, Rorschach, and the Bender must now be supplemented by interest surveys such as the Strong and particular aptitude studies.

An approach to the demented patient through psychological testing is exemplified by the case of a 27-year-old man whose behavior changed after an automobile accident. He had been comatose for several days after injury, which had occurred a year before testing. He had additionally become hypoxic, required tracheostomy, and experienced tentorial herniation. When he regained consciousness, his left limbs were weak, and he remained agitated, amnesic, and delirious for weeks. He was later regarded by his family as excessively talkative, his speech often being profane. Articulation and swallowing were impaired. He was emotionally volatile and labile. He had graduated from high school without distinction, married at an early age, and worked as a laborer at the time of the accident. His marriage, precipitated by his fiancee's pregnancy, had been marked by persistent instability and quarreling. His family believed that he had been indecisive and manifested impaired memory since regaining lucidity. He had been attempting to learn dental technology but was hampered by inability to retain the content of previous lessons. He had been forced to leave home owing to volatility and unrestrained anger. When he was referred for testing the psychologist was asked to: (1) estimate his original intelligence and quantify the degree of his dementia, (2) explore his capacities to remember, think, and make judgments, and (3) define his readiness for vocational training.

The psychologist used a clinical interview, the WAIS, Wechsler Memory Scale, Bender-Gestalt, and Rorschach Tests. On the WAIS, verbal I.Q. was 108 and performance I.Q. 106; his full-scale score of 108 indicated average intellectual function. Subtest analysis revealed inability to deal with proverbs, impaired abstract thinking, and poor control over associational processes. He did well when required to make short answers but became incoherent when longer responses were necessary. Visual motor organization was well preserved though the score on block design was lowest of the lot.

Because so many of his responses on the WAIS required intense effort, the Wechsler Memory Scale was administered. His memory quotient was 83 or "dull normal." He lost credit because of poor immediate recall of logical material and reproduction of geometric designs. His ability to learn new materials was impaired.

His reproductions of the figures on the Bender-Gestalt disclosed fairly good perception, but he had difficulty crossing lines, forming angles, and closing loops. These signs were regarded as consistent with "organic damage."

Projective testing (Rorschach and Bender-Gestalt) indicated reduced ability to form concepts, impaired associational processes, unstable controls, and a tendency to isolate parts of situations from the total. As a result, many of his conclusions bore little relevance to the total situation, and he was often uncritical of his judgments. This testing also disclosed him to be depressed about his disability and family problems. He attempted to deal with the latter by denial and compensation, but he became aggressive occasionally, especially when fatigued.

At about the same time, his capacity to operate a motor vehicle was evaluated in a driver trainer. His reaction times were generally slow; he had trouble complying with multiple commands; and his attitudes were described as "at the teenager level."

On the basis of these examinations the patient was judged to have significant deficits in judgment, emotional control, memory, and capacity to learn. His cognitive functions were little impaired. His driving test conformed to the conclusions drawn from psychological testing. Vocational training was held to be premature.

He was tested again 10 months later. There had been no change in his total WAIS score, but he achieved slightly higher scores in digit symbol and block design. His Wechsler Memory Scale disclosed marked improvement, from a previous score of 83 to 108, with improvement in immediate recall of logical material, reproduction of geometric designs, and ability to learn new material.

The improvement in memory function corresponded to increasing appropriateness in social behavior and ability to conform to the demands of a vocational training program in which he had enrolled.

Psychological testing may also assist the definition and direction of study of patients with evolving dementia but should not be a substitute for thorough clinical neurological evaluation. The common referral asks whether the process is organic or nonorganic, acute or chronic, focal or diffuse, stable or progressive, and associated or not with decompensation of previous personality patterns and intellectual functions.

A 47-year-old man illustrates the utilization of psychometry in the evaluation of an evolving illness. He was a retired army officer who had completed 3 years of college. In the months before examination he developed back pain and was found to have glycosuria. He became moody, worried, suspicious, and often failed to remember recent events and plans. Grasp reflexes, kinetic apraxia, fluctuating disorientation for time and space, impaired ability to abstract, frequent misidentification of persons, confabulation and distractibility were found on neurological examination. He often recognized his errors and wept in rage when he could not control or understand them. He was regarded as demented rather than depressed and was believed to suffer frontal lobe disease. Spinal fluid studies were normal, but the brain scan disclosed a poorly defined area of subfrontal midline uptake. The patient was referred with the following questions: (1) Is there organic disease? (2) Are the changes acute? (3) Is there evidence of focal or lateralized disease? (4) What prior personality patterns influence the clinical picture?

The tests selected in the first sessions were limited by his short attention span and concentrated on memory and visuomotor performance. These included the Bender-Gestalt Test, the Wechsler Memory Scale, and the Draw a Person Test. The results confirmed mental and intellectual deterioration, confabulation, concrete thinking, memory loss, and reduced new learning. Thus, the organic character of the disorder was substantiated. The degree of confusion, his volatility of mood, and the occasionally accurate test responses suggested an acute process. He retained rather good ability in calculation and was able to recite the alphabet accurately, count backward from 20 to 1 in 7 seconds, and from 1 to 40 by threes in 17 seconds. The Bender figures were constructed without gross distortion of form but with considerable looseness of lines and carelessness, indicating defective motor coordination and judgment. One figure provoked him to a tangential thought as he asked, "Are those starsies?" (little stars). Attempts to draw a person were similarly marked by difficulty controlling the line and gross variability so that the hair was drawn straight on one side and curly on the other. The patient numbered his efforts on the Bender-Gestalt Test, pointing to a previously compulsive and self-critical man.

The psychometrist concluded that the disturbance of complex intellectual activity with preservation of simple operations and the poorly controlled though not spatially distorted Bender figures pointed to frontal disease without lateralization. The test results were regarded as compatible with the clinical impression of presenile dementia or Pick's disease.

His behavioral disorder slowly intensified. At the second examination 3 months later he was more amenable, and the WAIS was added to his previous testing. His score was 97 (verbal 103 and performance 89). Picture completion, block design, comprehension, and digit span were the lowest of the subtest scores. The examiner now noted difficulties in strictly verbal tests and suggested a beginning aphasic disorder. The previous test results were little altered.

The second testing confirmed the previous finding of organic disease probably involving frontal lobes, but the suggested difficulty with language pointed to left frontal disease rather than diffuse bifrontal disease. Subsequently a subfrontal dermoid cyst, which involved the medial surface of both frontal lobes but more extensively affected the left, was removed. In this case, testing assisted by confirming the organic and relatively acutely progressive character of the disorder, by identifying the prior personality patterns, and ultimately by hinting accurately at correct cerebral localization.

Identification and quantification of dementia may be difficult for the physician and psychologist when the defects are subtle, particularly when associated with apparently neurotic symptoms. In such cases, anxiety, paranoia, or depression may accompany the evolving dementia. *As a general rule the less definitive the results of searching clinical neurological assessment, the less clear will be the results of psychological study.* The common early signs of dementia on psychological testing involve visual motor disorders, loss of ability to shift from one form of reference to another, impaired memory, and reduced capacities for synthesis, generalization, and organization. These are usually reflected in impaired performance rather than in verbal tests. The WAIS may be entirely normal except for slight and selective impairment in digit symbol and reversal of digits on the digit span tests. The Bender-Gestalt Test may disclose some clumsiness in construction, especially of complex interlocking figures, perseveration, rotation of figures, and fragmentation of design. These may be the earliest signs detected by psychological testing. The Rorschach may be abnormal owing to slowness, reduced number of responses, and preoccupation with detail. The Wechsler Memory Scale may disclose additional evidence of impaired memory and new learning. The Goldstein-Scheerer Test and Halstead or Reitan batteries may amplify impaired abstracting ability.

If the patient has little awareness of his difficulty, denial and projection are frequent findings with the projective techniques. Alternatively, patients who are aware in some way of their deficits though unable to compensate for them may respond with depression or anxiety. Previous personality patterns appear to be heightened. Repeated evaluations of such patients disclose that the "minimal signs of organicity" become increasingly specific as total intellectual function becomes affected by evolving disease.

A retired contractor became depressed, anxious, and preoccupied as his limbs became weak and his voice hoarse. He cried easily and often quarreled with people, contrary to his usual custom. His family and physician denied loss of intellectual function, attributing to depression symptoms such as loss of train of thought, impaired naming, and inability to find common properties in similar objects. On psychological study all tests indicated organic impairment, but tests of conceptualization such as similarity on the WAIS were strikingly impaired though arithmetic was preserved. The digit span was but five numbers forward. He could not accommodate to reversal. Block design was very poor. At his death he was found to have sustained widespread neuronal degeneration.

Planning care for a patient with manifest disease of the brain may require knowledge of the premorbid intellectual state and estimation of possible interference with behavior by an accompanying emotional reaction. Sometimes intertest analysis is helpful in this determination.

A 26-year-old man sustained a gunshot wound of the right parietal region. The bullet had crossed the central midline and lay in his left occipital lobe. He was totally blind save for a small island in the upper temporal quadrant of the left visual field, where he could name objects, identify colors, and read some words. His right side was weak. Position sense was impaired bilaterally, more so on the left. Tactile localization, response to double simultaneous stimulation, and stereognosis were impaired in the left limbs. Auditory localization favored the right side of space. There was impaired sentence formation, naming, and repetition. Paraphasia was present. A psychological evaluation was required in planning mobility training.

The verbal portion of the WAIS was used. The verbal score was 78, but scores on information, similarities, comprehension, and vocabulary were 9 or 10, indicating that his premorbid intelligence was within normal range. His mood was stable during examination and not depressed. The high scores on the tests listed above indicated preserved reasoning, judgment, and concept formation. The psychometrist noted syntactical difficulty and perseveration. Immediate memory was markedly impaired as shown by a score of but one point on digit span. He scored zero on arithmetic. Thus, tasks requiring prolonged concentration and attention and change of mental set were too difficult for him.

These observations confirmed the clinical opinion that the patient was not ready for mobility training and that his behavior did not result from a psychological reaction to injury.

NEUROPSYCHOLOGICAL METHODS

Tests of intelligence, cognition, personality, and aptitude are performed in most clinical settings and are adequate for most purposes. More detailed neuropsychological study of specific mental impairment is becoming increasingly available as a clinical tool and offers opportunities to study sensation, vision, memory, motor skills, hemispheric dominance, and language competence in ways not hitherto available, as well as affording tools for the experimental study of human behavior.

Flicker-fusion frequency in the quadrants of the visual field may be determined as an adjunct to standard perimetry and may disclose abnormalities associated with posterior superior parietal disorders when changes on standard perimetric examination are minor or inapparent. When fusion frequencies are reduced, *apparent motion* is less well perceived in the affected visual sectors. The *capacity to perceive figures* upon brief tachistoscopic exposure or to reverse a cube or other figure may also be abnormal, though with less localizing value.

Somatosensory disorders are often associated with inability to draw complete human figures, clock faces, or identify body sides or parts. *Visual disorientation in the dimensions of space* may be shown by inability to localize objects in space, bisect lines, or arrange objects in three dimensions. Patterns of ocular search may be recorded by means of special photographic equipment. The *time required for searching localization* may be measured by asking the patient to hunt in a field of objects one that resembles another placed in the center. In all these studies it is possible to search for general as well as lateralized or quadrantic somatosensory or visuospatial disorders. The studies have their major applicability in cases of unilateral or bilateral parietal disorder.

The temporal lobe's auditory functions have only recently begun to be the subject of extensive study. Tests of tonality, pitch, threshold, and musical ability are not extensively employed except as part of the Halstead battery (q.v.). Learning and memory can be shown to be affected after severe temporal lesions that do not render the patient aphasic. While the total score obtained on Wechsler Memory Scale may be reduced, the greatest impairment in recall of verbal material is said to occur after 1 to 2 hours' lapse. Failures have been described as particularly pronounced following left temporal lesions. Comprehension of pictorial abnormalities appears to be disproportionately impaired by right temporal lesions and has been measured by means of the McGill Picture Abnormalities Test, which consists of sketches containing ridiculous situations that the patient is to identify. Maze learning has been used as a special memory test. The tests require the subject to discover, learn, and remember a complex pattern. Other memory tests ask the patient to remember such compound stimuli as successive tones or clicks for periods of up to 1 minute by indicating whether a second signal is identical to the first.

Batteries of tests have been designed to study the effects of frontal lobe disease. They include form and figure matching and recall, flicker-fusion frequency in the central visual field, finger tapping, sorting and categorization tests, and definition and differentiation of words.

Reitan has applied a comprehensive group of tests to study the effects of cerebral disease on behavior and to predict the nature and locus of the disorder. His battery consists of the WAIS, Halstead's neuropsychological tests, a modification of the Halstead-Wepman Aphasia Screening Test, the Minnesota Multiphasic Personality Inventory, Reitan's Trailmaking Test, and tests of sensory and perceptual function.

The Halstead battery of ten tests is directed toward the discovery of frontal lobe disease. The Category Test requires the subject to discern relationships among visually presented objects by hypothesis formation and adapt these concepts to further problem solving as reinforcement accompanies correct responses. The test is nonverbal and depends upon such factors as size, shape, and color of the components. It is regarded as a test of abstraction ability and attempts to quantify this function. In the Halstead battery, flicker-fusion is used in the central field where reduced frequency is said to relate to frontal lobe disorder. The Tactual Performance Test compares the rapidity with which a blindfolded patient replaces forms in a formboard using either and both hands. Memory for the number, shape, and localization of the parts of the board is tested by asking the patient to sketch it. The Seashore Test of Musical Talent requires the patient to discriminate among rhythm sequences and depends upon alertness and attention. The latter are also required on the Speech Sounds Perception Test as the patient must match spoken sounds to letters on a board. The Finger Oscillation Test requires the subject to activate a mechanical counter at maximum speed for 10 seconds with the index finger of either hand. The Time Sense Test first requires the patient to start a clock and then stop it in the starting position after 10 seconds while looking at it. After ten trials he is required to repeat the performance blindfolded. An "impairment index" derived from the components of the Halstead battery is said to identify patients with frontal lobe impairment.

The Halstead-Wepman Aphasia Screening Test surveys systematically such language attributes as naming, spelling, articulation, reading, writing, and comprehension.

The Trailmaking Test requires the patient first to connect numbered circles in ascending sequence and then to alternate between numerical and alphabetical circles.

Sensoriperceptual tests include double simultaneous tactile, auditory, and visual stimulation, tactile finger recognition, tactile form recognition in each hand, and perception of numbers written on the tips of the fingers of each hand.

Such advanced neuropsychological testing is time consuming, complex, and requires skilled personnel. Many such as the Category Test attempt to quantify the process of abstraction, which, along with other mental processes, has hitherto been only described and identified. The superiority of such neuropsychological study over the combination of clinical neurological examination augmented by selective psychological testing and other laboratory procedures has yet to be proved.

SUMMARY OF THE FINDINGS IN FOCAL AND DIFFUSE DISEASE

Though the clinical need for psychological tests accurate in identifying diffuse, lateralized, or focal disease of the brain has led to expansion of neuropsychological procedures available, many of these are used in but a few centers. This discussion is therefore limited to widely used clinical tests and is intended as a guide for the physician. (See Table 1.) Since psychological testing

Table I. Psychological testing in dementia

Condition	Tests and Anticipated Results	Clinical Comments
Questionable or minimal dementia with or without neurotic features	WAIS: Impairment may be minor except for digits backward and digit symbol. Bender-Gestalt: Slight clumsiness, distortion of size, shape, rotation, displacement. Goldstein-Scheerer: Impaired ability to abstract and shift mental set. Wechsler Memory Scale: Immediate recall, new learning reduced.	Variations in Wechsler subtests may be insufficient to lower total score but become significant when combined with other measures. Inferences of organic deficit may depend upon individualization of testing and the use of non-quantifiable measures, clinical interview, and history. Neurotic features (anxiety, compulsivity, depression, denial) may distort organic signs.
Manifest dementia secondary to a widespread process, e.g., the effects of hypertensive cerebrovascular disease or hypoxia, Alzheimer's disease	WAIS: Total score lowered. Verbal higher than performance. Digit span, digit symbol, block design usually maximally involved. Arithmetic, similarities, object assembly less so. Vocabulary well preserved. Bender-Gestalt: Quite abnormal with distorted figures, over-sized or undersized, displaced upward on page, many corrections, figures simplified or fragmented. Rorschach: Responses reduced in number, slow, fragmentary, concrete.	Usually easily identified, findings correspond to those on physical examination. Useful for documentation and following rate of progression. Test results highly sensitive to medication, hypoxia, hypoglycemia, fatigue, fever, and metabolic derangement.
Mental deficiency	WAIS: Total score low. Arithmetic, digits backward, digit symbol, block design low. Object assembly, vocabulary and comprehension may be higher than average subtest score.	Subtest scores may be quite uniform. Digits backward invariably affected. High arithmetic and block design scores incompatible with clinical diagnosis. Testing vulnerable to emotional disorder.
Dementia associated with gross focal pathology		As a clinical rule dementia attributable to a unilateral cerebral lesion is invariably associated with gross signs such as hemiplegia or hemianesthesia.
Bifrontal lobe disease	WAIS may be little affected. Digit reversal and similarities impaired when attention and concentration are. Color-form, object sorting (Goldstein-Scheerer), new learning, logical memory (Wechsler Memory Scale) impaired.	Reasoning and problem solving usually impaired. Testing may require individualization. If available the Halstead or Reitan battery is useful, especially Category Test, Flicker-Fusion, and Finger Tapping. Depression may appear on projective tests.

Location		
Right frontal	A most difficult area to specify until disease is extensive. Left hemiparesis or left grasp reflex usually detectable.	Color-form, object sorting slightly impaired. Tests of motor performance with left hand slow.
Left frontal	Aphasia screening and finger oscillation tests (right or both hands) abnormal. Constructional tests relatively spared.	Verbal tests on WAIS may be impaired along with digit reversal, digit symbol. Blocks less so. Abstracting loss seen on color-form, object sorting. Difficulty writing on Bender, manipulating cards on Rorschach. Responses reduced in number and highly concrete; language agrammatical on Rorschach.
Bitemporal (sparing left lateral temporal lobe)	Memory and orientation markedly affected. Any test of memory likely to be sensitive indicator. Confabulation and disorientation, especially on clinical interview, prominent in recent lesions, e.g., Korsakoff's disease. When lateral portions left temporal lobe involved, language impaired.	Digit span, digit reversal, digit symbol particularly impaired on the WAIS though conspicuous performance and verbal defects may be present. New learning, reproduction of stories, memory for figures grossly impaired on all tests.
Right temporal	Maze learning, tests of time sense, McGill Picture Abnormalities abnormal and useful when available. Tests of language normal. Reasoning little impaired. The process affected here is memory for visually presented material.	Picture completion, object assembly, block design reduced on WAIS. Some distortion, rotation, neglect of one side on Bender-Gestalt. Rorschach responses often from right side of card.
Left temporal	Halstead, Reitan batteries often abnormal when tests of tonality, pitch, threshold, and aphasia screening are used. Memory for verbally presented material, naming, language comprehension most affected. Should be evident on clinical examination.	Performance portion on WAIS usually better than verbal components. Recall of verbal material on Wechsler Memory Scale markedly abnormal. Naming on WAIS (e.g., picture completion) and Rorschach may be abnormal. Syntactical errors and paraphasia in spoken speech.
Biparietal	Visuomotor, visual perceptual abnormalities readily detected by most standard measures. Projective techniques may disclose denial, hallucinosis, projection. These tests combined with aphasia screening, sorting and abstraction help identify left frontal, parietal processes.	WAIS performance items highly abnormal, especially block design, digit symbol, object assembly. Rorschach: no or few highly concrete perseverated responses. Bender-Gestalt figures simplified, displaced upward, fragmented, incorrectly proportioned. Draw a Person shows similar distortions.

Table 1. Continued

Condition	Tests and Anticipated Results	Clinical Comments
Right parietal	WAIS performance items resemble above. Right-left confusion or preoccupation with right side seen on picture completion, object assembly, or picture arrangement. Rorschach responses may be exclusively from right side of card often with highly unusual figure completion or confabulation. Bender figures abnormal with marked distortion, rotation, and neglect of left side.	Readily detected by standard measures. "Sensoriperceptual" tests of Reitan battery invariably abnormal and indicate right parietal lesion. Denial, projection, delusions may be prominent. Use of language may be concrete though not aphasic.
Left parietal	WAIS performance items better preserved than verbal. Arithmetic and digit span markedly impaired when testable. Picture completion may be abnormal. Digit symbol may be impossible for the patient to do. Bender, Rorschach may be beyond patient's comprehension. Bender figures usually highly simplified. Aphasia screening tests abnormal, with respect to reading, writing. Goldstein-Scheerer abnormal, especially cube and object sorting.	Sensoriperceptual tests on Reitan usually indicate impaired perception of numbers written on fingertip and tactile form recognition bilaterally. WAIS performance items often beetter preserved than when right parietal lobe involved.
Bioccipital	Visual testing impossible. Nonvisual testing, especially form recognition and memory, and verbal portion of WAIS usually normal.	Patient aware of blindness and compensates for it. With acute lesion invariably seriously depressed. Parieto-occipital lesions usually associated with denial and blindness, hallucinosis and erratic tactile form recognition, memory, similarities, and arithmetic.
Right, left occipital	Compensated lesions should not affect testing. Uncompensated ones are associated with neglect of one side and constructional errors resembling parietal lesions.	Pure unilateral occipital lesion uncommon. Hemianopia usually adequately compensated. A rare patient with para-callosal lesion is unable to read with right homonymous hemianopia.

measures mental processes, the results should always be interpreted in terms of disturbance of function and only secondarily in terms of anatomical loci or pathological processes. Disturbance of psychological function may or may not be indicative of structural lesions of the brain. Moreover, one should remind himself that "isolated" disturbances of psychological function are rare indeed and that opinions relative to focal and diffuse disease are derived by combining several positive and negative pieces of information.

In patients suffering widespread brain disease all major functions may be depressed. Constructions will be found simplified, motor control impaired, memory shortened, and abstracting ability grossly reduced. Sensitive indicators on the WAIS include block design, digit symbol, similarities, picture arrangement, and picture completion. Bender figures will be poorly reproduced, clumsily drawn, and often crowded to the top of the page. Considerable perseveration may be encountered. On Rorschach testing the totality and rate of response are reduced, and the patient is usually preoccupied with detail rather than with integration of the whole. Memory and new learning are grossly impaired on the Wechsler Memory Scale with digit span (especially backward) showing the greatest impairment.

"Diffuse" brain disease may take on regional characteristics. In frontal lobe disease certain simple mental functions may be retained, including arithmetic, digit retention forward, vocabulary, or information, but when abstraction, generalization, or the performance of complex tasks is tested, the loss becomes evident. Thus, tests of similarity on the WAIS (e.g., the common property of a seed and egg) and generalization (the Goldstein-Scheerer or other sorting test) may be grossly abnormal. Impaired motor control on visual motor tests (Draw a Person or Bender-Gestalt) is shown by careless and inaccurate drawing though the shapes of the figures are not distorted.

Processes maximally affecting the parietal lobes usually produce their most striking changes in cognitive processes. These may be seen on the WAIS by impairment in such visually directed performance measures as block design, picture completion, digit symbol, and arithmetic. Relative preservation of vocabulary, comprehension, and information is usual. On constructional tests, such as the Bender-Gestalt and Draw a Person, figures tend to be grossly simplified. Irregular pentagons may become squares and complex figures fragmented into components. The position of figures relative to one another becomes distorted or rotated. Human figures lose detail and their form becomes regular, e.g., round rather than oval. There may be only a few highly concrete Rorschach responses.

Temporal lobe disorders that spare language function are usually characterized by severe memory loss, inattentiveness, and impairment of new learning. Constructions are usually well done. Items on the WAIS that depend upon the patient's remembering a task and completing it are grossly impaired. Hence, digit symbol, digit span, arithmetic, and picture arrangement may be

77

markedly abnormal. Block design and picture completion may be less affected, and vocabulary, information, and comprehension relatively spared. The Wechsler Memory Scale discloses extreme impairment in recent and remote memory and in new learning. Visual motor performance on the Bender-Gestalt and Draw a Person tests is relatively well preserved. Nonetheless, in this situation as with other forms of regional but bilateral brain disease, the bias of influence upon specific psychological performance is only relative, and total performance is invariably impaired.

Clinical psychological testing is most helpful when it calls attention to a clinical or lateralizing phenomenon not previously detected. The concept of the localization of psychic mental function in man revolves around the specialization of the left cerebrum for speech. When the left frontal lobe is affected, a disorder of speech may be reflected in the purely verbal portions of the WAIS, which may be disproportionately involved. When the patient uses language on the Rorschach, Bender-Gestalt, or Draw a Person Tests, language errors may also appear. Frequently apractic agraphia in the absence of weakness may be evident on the Bender-Gestalt and other constructional tests.

A lesion affecting the left temporal and parietal lobes is inevitably associated with some disorder of language function, often severe enough to preclude extensive testing owing to failure of comprehension or articulation. When examination is possible, a mixture of constructional, performance, and language difficulties may be encountered. On the WAIS, verbal tests and digit symbol may be untestable. Block design, picture completion, arithmetic, similarities and reversal of digit span (when testable) may be impaired. The Bender figures may be crowded to the left side of the page, greater emphasis being given to the left side of figures with many of the gestalten simplified. Thus, five-sided figures may be reproduced as squares and intersecting lines of tangential figures separated from one another. There may also be rotation of figures so that their horizontal axis slants downward to the right. (By contrast, when the lesion is right sided the inclination is often upward and to the right.) Erasures, scratching out, and drawing over errors are often absent, in contrast to their prominence with lesions elsewhere. The number of Rorschach responses is greatly reduced or absent. When present they tend to be fragmentary and may be perceived from the left side of the card. The Wechsler Memory Scale may disclose marked impairment for learning and recalling verbally presented material. The Wechsler Memory Scale, verbal and picture completion portions of the WAIS, and the Rorschach Tests may also disclose striking paraphasia, impaired naming, or the substitution of cognate words. When the balance of impairment is toward verbally presented material, the lesion is thought to be relatively laterally placed, i.e., toward the temporal lobe. When constructional, arithmetic, and visual impairments are more pronounced, the lesion is regarded as more parietal. Parietotemporal lesions of the left hemisphere usually produce the most striking defects of all focal lesions, probably reflecting the verbal character of the tests and of human intellectual activity.

When disease is preponderant in the right parietotemporal region, construc--tional disorders may appear most prominently affected on tests of figure drawing and the Bender-Gestalt. The right side of the figure usually receives greater emphasis, and drawings may be crowded toward the right side of the page. Similar neglect on the left side may appear in tests involving reading a line, e.g., the digit symbol and picture arrangement portions of the WAIS, and in preoccupation with the right side of Rorschach cards. Block design may be impossible. Occasionally these defects are so evident to the psychometrist that he may even demonstrate a visual field defect by confrontation testing. Impairment of visual recognition may affect tests such as picture completion. Such conditions are believed to result from involvement on the right temporal lobe's lateral convexity. Many of the neuropsychological techniques discussed above, including critical flicker-fusion frequency, tactile localization, and double simultaneous tactile stimulation, can be appropriately employed here.

Purely occipital disorders are uncommon. They cause relatively little specific change other than inattentiveness to one side of space (opposite to the cerebral lesion), and even this is not striking.

Right frontal lesions per se may be very difficult to identify, and anticipated disorders of judgment and planning, as might be shown by the Bender-Gestalt or tests of abstraction such as the Goldstein-Scheerer, may be inconclusive until the lesion is quite large and general effects appear.

The manner in which focal cerebral lesions influence test function depends to a large part upon the degree to which the tests involve language and verbal comprehension. The more verbal the test and the instructions, the more likely it is that left cerebral lesions will impair test results out of proportion to comparable right-sided lesions. Conversely, right-sided lesions that do not alter language comprehension will have their greatest effect on performance items such as block design and figure construction. Additionally, postrolandic left-sided lesions produce greater defects than do comparable ones elsewhere in the left hemisphere. *Test results in cases of focal lesions are likely to be abnormal in the following order: left temporal and parietal, left frontal and occipital, right temporal and parietal, right occipital and right frontal.*

One should recall Wechsler's admonition, however, that function is invariably globally involved even though distinctive patterns may be evident and that any lesion large enough to disrupt "local" function also has a general disintegrative effect. The degree and pattern of dissolution of intellectual function do not necessarily reflect an immutable anatomically determined alteration.

REFERENCES

1. BENDER, L.: *A visual motor Gestalt test and its clinical use.* Res. Monogr. Amer. Orthopsychiat. Assn. No. 3, 1938.

2. DARLEY, J. G., AND HAGENAH, T.: *Vocational Interest Measurement, Theory, and Practice.* University of Minnesota Press, Minneapolis, 1955.

3. GOLDSTEIN, K., AND SCHEERER, M.: *Abstract and concrete behavior: An experimental study with special tests.* Psychol. Monogr. 53:2, 1941.

4. GOLDSTEIN, K., AND SCHEERER, M.: *Goldstein-Scheerer Test of Abstract and Concrete Thinking.* Physiological Corporation, New York, 1945.

5. HALSTEAD, W. C.: *Brain and Intelligence.* University of Chicago Press, Chicago, 1947.

6. HALSTEAD, W. C.: Brain and intelligence, in Jeffress, L. A. (ed.) : *Cerebral Mechanisms in Behavior: The Hixson Symposium.* John Wiley & Sons, New York, 1951.

7. HATHAWAY, S. R., AND McKINLEY, J. C.: *The Minnesota Multiphasic Personality Inventory.* University of Minnesota Press, Minneapolis, 1942.

8. KLOPFER, B., AINSWORTH, M., KLOPFER, W. G., AND HOLD, R. R.: *Developments in the Rorschach Technique. I. Technique and Theory.* World Book Co., Yonkers, 1954.

9. KLOPFER, B., AND KELLY, D. M.: *The Rorschach Technique.* World Book Co., Yonkers, 1942.

10. LURIA, A. R.: *Neuropsychology in the local diagnosis of brain damage.* Cortex 1:3, 1964.

11. MURRAY, H. A.: *Thematic Apperception Test.* Harvard University Press, Cambridge, Mass., 1943.

12. PASCAL, G., AND SUTTELL, B. J.: *The Bender-Gestalt Test: Its Quantification and Validity for Adults.* Grune & Stratton, New York, 1951.

13. REITAN, R. M.: *Problems and prospects in studying the psychological correlates of brain lesions.* Cortex 2:127, 1966.

14. REITAN, R. M.: A research program on the psychological effects of brain lesions in human beings, in Ellis, N. R. (ed.) : *International Review of Research in Mental Retardation.* Academic Press, New York, 1966.

15. RORSCHACH, H.: *Psychodiagnostics. A Diagnostic Test Based on Perception.* Grune & Stratton, New York, 1942.

16. TEUBER, H-L.: Neuropsychology, in Harrower, M. R. (ed.) : *Recent Advances in Diagnostic Psychological Testing.* Charles C Thomas, Publisher, Springfield, Ill., 1950.

17. TOMKINS, S. S., HORN, D., AND MINER, J. B.: *The Tomkins-Horn Picture Arrangement Test.* Springer Publishing Co., Inc., New York, 1957.

18. WECHSLER, D.: *The Measurement and Appraisal of Adult Intelligence,* ed. 4. The Williams & Wilkins Co., Baltimore, 1958.

Chapter 5

The Electroencephalogram
in Dementia*

M. J. Short, M.D., and
W. P. Wilson, M.D.

* From the Division of Clinical Neurophysiology of the Department of Psychiatry, Duke University Medical Center, Durham, North Carolina.

In the clinical evaluation of dementia, electroencephalography is a useful, physiologically based tool to extend the clinical examination. It is simple, easy to apply, and repeatable, which allows its use both in diagnosis and in assessment of progression of a disease process. It is therefore an essential part of the accessory examination of the demented patient.[21]

In evaluating the electroencephalogram (EEG), it is useful to follow the evaluation suggested by Cobb[5] based on (1) the frequency and amplitude of its rhythmic components; (2) the location, distribution, and hemispheric symmetry of its rhythmic and transient components; (3) the form of the rhythmic and transient components; and (4) their reactivity to commonly used activating techniques, including eye opening, hyperventilation, intermittent photic stimulation, and sleep. The response to each of the procedures carries with it a degree of diagnostic significance and prognostic value.

NORMAL AGING

Since the development of the EEG, there have been many reports correlating electroencephalographic findings with the clinical condition of the aged patient. The first report on the application of the EEG in dementia was made in 1939 by Rubin.[45] His analysis focused upon changes in "per cent time alpha," i.e., the percentage of time that the alpha rhythm is present in an EEG record in patients with dementia. In eight of nine patients, a decreased per cent time alpha correlated with pneumoencephalographic evidence of unilateral hemispherical atrophy.

Changes in alpha rhythms have served as one of the basic parameters in EEG evaluation of conditions associated with dementia. In his pioneering investigation on EEG and aging, Davis[6] demonstrated a slowing of the alpha frequency with a decreasing alpha index (equivalent to per cent time alpha expressed in decimals) accompanied by increased slow activity (Fig. 1). This study was made on aging neuropsychiatric patients. It was not until 1953 that an EEG investigation was carried out on a group of normal old people to contrast and supplement the earlier reports[17,25,26,29] on abnormal EEG's in senile patients. In a study of 329 persons over 60 years of age, Busse and associates[4] noted much variation in the EEG's of psychologically normal old people. In fact, they found both normal and abnormal EEG's. There was a tendency for the basic background frequencies to decrease. Their most frequent observation was the presence of focal theta, particularly in the left anterior temporal region, not correlated with cerebral dominance. This focal abnormality increased with increasing years. When pathological change due to cerebral vascular disease was present, the slow activity was general rather than focal.

The work of Obrist[38] not only corroborates the observation of Busse and his group[4] but extends our comprehension of the variety of EEG findings in healthy older persons. Obrist noted that the mean occipital alpha frequency shifts from 11 to 12 hertz (Hz) in middle-aged persons to 7 to 8 Hz in persons

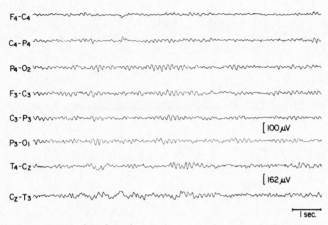

F4-C4

C4-P4

P4-O2

F3-C3

C3-P3

[100 μV

P3-O1

T4-Cz

[162 μV

Cz-T3

1 sec.

Figure I. A 78-year-old female with normal mental function. The EEG demonstrates slowing of the alpha frequency to 7 and 7½ Hz. There is also bitemporal slowing, which is a common finding in this age group without clinical significance or correlation.

in their senium with an accompanying reduction in the alpha index. Focal slowing occurred in the temporo-occipital region in 4 per cent of normal aged males, while 8 per cent showed bilateral synchronous slowing in the fronto-parietal region and 2 per cent had bilateral independent slowing. Obrist also observed that the response to hyperventilation was either minimal or absent in the EEG of older individuals.

In summary, the electrical activity of the brain changes with age, whether or not there is clinically recognizable cerebral disease. The typical EEG changes of the senium are decreasing frequency of alpha rhythm, lower per cent time alpha, unilateral temporal slowing or symmetrical anterior slowing, and decreased sensitivity of hyperventilation.[13,30,51]

SENILE DEMENTIA

The altered electroencephalographic pattern found in some mentally normal aged individuals is accentuated in conditions associated with loss of the mental faculties. Davis and Davis[7] stated that "although the psychotic individual cannot be recognized by his EEG, nevertheless as a group the psychotics have a significantly larger percentage of abnormalities in their EEG's than do normals." In the study by Mundy-Castle and his co-workers[35] of 50 mentally normal senile persons and 104 patients with senile psychosis, 24 per cent of the normal group had abnormal EEG's whereas 44 per cent of the senile psychotic group had abnormal EEG's. The characteristic abnormality was diffuse slowing to theta (Fig. 2) and even delta frequencies (Fig. 3). These authors identified a significant relationship between increasing dementia and the presence of increased diffuse theta activity and reduced alpha index. A significant re-

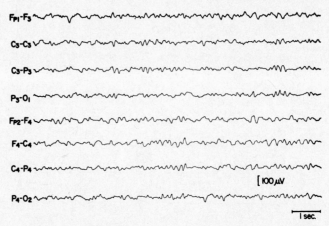

Figure 2. A 73-year-old patient with senile dementia whose EEG is generally slowed in all head regions. Cerebral background rhythms are poorly developed.

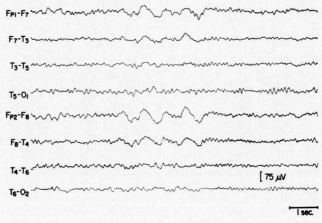

Figure 3. A 71-year-old female with intermittent slowing bilaterally in the central regions. This is a common EEG abnormality in patients with senile dementia. There is also intermittent slowing of the alpha rhythm to less than 8 Hz.

duction of beta activity was also observed. These results are in accord with earlier reports by McAdam and McClatchey.[30]

Weiner and Schuster[57] reported that the pattern of abnormal slow activity in senile dementia is predominantly nonfocal, either diffuse or scattered, and is not a seizure-burst type of discharge. Increased low-voltage paroxysmal fast (LVF) activity is prominent in normal old persons but infrequent in patients with senile dementia, although it does occur (Fig. 4). Weiner and Schuster further recognized a strong correlation between the severity of EEG involvement and the degree of dementia. Similar observations have been made by

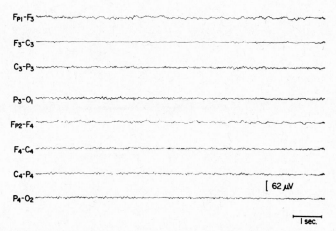

Figure 4. A 67-year-old female with classical senile dementia. The EEG demonstrates a low-voltage fast record with generalized slowing, an infrequent finding in senile dementia.

Short, Musella, and Wilson,[50] who demonstrated a curvilinear relation of EEG abnormalities to both mentation and affection in senile patients. This finding would lead one to expect a number of normal records in patients in the early phases of the illness. This is in contrast to the report of McAdam and Robinson,[31] who identified a linear relationship between the clinical level of intellectual impairment and EEG involvement.

There is good correlation between encephalographic abnormalities and

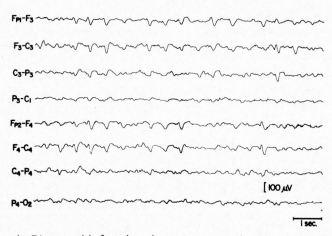

Figure 5. A 71-year-old female who presents with dementia. The EEG is characterized by triphasic waves that appear bilaterally in the anterior head regions. Laboratory evaluations demonstrated compromised liver function with hyperammonemia.

nonfocal cerebral atrophy in senile dementia. Low-voltage fast-frequency records, common in normal aged persons, are uncommon in patients with dilated ventricles. When convulsive seizures occurred in the presence of cortical atrophy or ventricular dilation, the EEG was invariably abnormal.[24,53] The correlation between EEG findings and cerebral atrophy has been borne out by brain scanning.[36]

Muller and Kral[34] correlated the occurrence of bilaterally synchronous slow wave discharges of a triphasic character (similar to those seen in hepatic coma) with advanced senile and presenile psychoses without alteration of consciousness (Fig. 5). The prognosis in these patients was quite poor, prompting the "malignant" senile amnestic syndrome classification. In our own laboratories, however, we have found that almost all of the patients with triphasic waves have liver failure with hyperammonemia.

PRESENILE DEMENTIA

The abiotrophic theory[15] of presenile dementia anticipates EEG findings in these conditions qualitatively similar and probably quantitatively worse than those abnormalities seen in senile dementia. In 17 cases of pathologically verified Alzheimer's disease, Letemendia and Pampiglione[23] found generalized 2 to 7 Hz activity, which responded minimally to external stimuli. There was, however, a paradoxical increase in frequency with hyperventilation and drowsiness. Sleep spindles were recognizable but were of low voltage. The degree of EEG abnormality correlated uniformly with the severity of the dementia. Further observations on EEG changes in Alzheimer's disease were made by Liddell.[27] In contrast to the authors cited, he characterized the EEG patterns of Alzheimer's disease as having "a generalized basic rhythm of diffuse medium amplitude theta or slow alpha activity at 6 to 8 cycles per second (cps). Superimposed on this basic activity, paroxysmal bursts of synchronous high amplitude delta waves occurred. These bursts had a tendency to repeat themselves rhythmically and were of greatest amplitude in the frontal and temporal regions." During barbiturate-induced sleep, the spontaneous K complexes of light sleep became absent and paroxysmal delta was abolished. Liddell did not correlate the degree of EEG involvement with the severity of the dementia.

In a longitudinal EEG study of the three major presenile dementia states—Alzheimer's, Pick's, and Jakob-Creutzfeldt's diseases—Gordon and Sim[14] found no differential components of dementia for the assessment of clinical-EEG relationships. The important factor when interpreting EEG's was to take into account the stage of the dementing process. Their findings demonstrated a reduction or absence of alpha rhythm, often with a concomitant flattening of the record, in the early stages of dementia. Later, low to medium voltage theta and delta discharges appeared rhythmically or diffusely (Fig. 6). Focal abnormalities were rarely present.

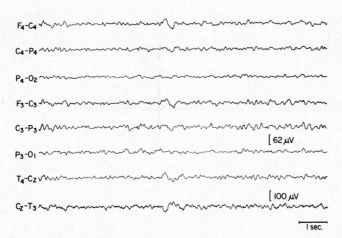

Figure 6. A 60-year-old female with a 3-year history of cerebral degenerative disease diagnosed at autopsy as Pick's disease. The EEG is characterized by the absence of alpha rhythm and the presence of theta and delta activity occurring symmetrically in the central regions and bitemporally.

Thus, many variables contribute to the alteration of EEG's in presenile dementia. One of the most consistent observations is the absence of the low-voltage fast-frequency records common in elderly persons. Secondly, there is reduction of the frequency of alpha rhythm in presenile dementia. The appearance of slow wave activity, initially in the theta frequency and subsequently in the delta range, provides additional evidence of cerebral involvement. Slow activity usually appears superimposed on the background rhythms, coming in paroxysmal bursts in the frontal and temporal regions.

Jakob-Creutzfeldt's disease exhibits a succession of EEG changes that have been of considerable interest to neurologists and electroencephalographers. Abbott[1] first aroused this interest by his description in two patients of regularly recurring diffuse high-voltage sharp waves (up to $350\mu v$), with first slowing, then flattening of the background activity between the sharp wave discharges. Similar high-voltage triphasic sharp waves have been observed in a number of patients with Jakob-Creutzfeldt's disease, usually in its advanced stages in the presence of both changes in level of consciousness and myoclonic jerks. They have been indeed so consistent as to be called "pathognomonic" of the disorder.[11] Hoefer[18] strongly disputed this contention, however, and there can be little doubt that discharges indistinguishable from these have been observed in a variety of conditions.[22]

During the final stage of Jakob-Creutzfeldt's disease, Nelson[37] stereotactically placed depth electrodes in the midline and lateral thalamus, caudate nucleus, internal capsule, subcortical white matter, and upper reticular formation. Recording from these areas showed synchronous discharges occurring in the subcortical areas. He thus suggested that these discharges do not arise from the cortex but are volume-conducted potentials generated by a single source within the upper brainstem.

The studies in this disorder have been well summarized by May:[33]

> . . . the EEG in Creutzfeldt-Jakob disease may present various changes throughout the course of the illness. It may be normal in the presence of definite neurological abnormalities, initially and to the end. Usually, however, there is some diffuse or focal slowing which correlates with the clinical changes and which finally is succeeded by a very characteristic pattern of regular slow triphasic bursts superimposed on a progressively slow cortical background activity. This pattern . . . is . . . not pathognomonic of Creutzfeldt-Jakob disease. However, it is quite characteristic and may be helpful in the diagnosis, though only late in the course.

In contrast to the focal-to-diffuse involvement occurring in the other presenile states, Huntington's chorea demonstrates global cerebral cortical involvement electroencephalographically. The characteristic pattern for the EEG involves the absence of rhythmical background activity with low-voltage intermittent random activity of theta and delta frequencies. Alpha rhythm tends to be absent in the parieto-occipital region. As in other heredodegenerative states, there is either minimal or no change with hyperventilation in Huntington's chorea.[16]

Although Parkinson's disease, whether presenile or senile in origin, is not generally classified among the dementias, a significant portion of patients suffering from Parkinson's disease are found to be demented.[43] Patients with parkinsonism frequently have abnormal EEG's.[9,48,52] In the Duke Laboratories parkinsonian patients with dementia are almost always found to have a diffusely abnormal record. As well, there is a good correlation between the outcome of neurolytic surgery and the EEG,[52] an abnormal preoperative EEG often being associated with a failure of postoperative rehabilitation.

CEREBROVASCULAR DISEASE

The differentiation of generalized cerebral arteriosclerosis from senile dementia is difficult electroencephalographically, as pointed out by Obrist and Busse.[39] When evaluating the relation of the EEG to cerebral vascular disease, it should be kept in mind that the usual electrode array covers only 25 per cent of the cerebral cortex. The remainder is buried in depths of sulci and underneath the frontal, temporal, and occipital lobes. Thus, most routine EEG's record mainly the area of arterial supply of the middle cerebral artery. In addition, the EEG abnormality depends upon the quantity of infarcted tissue and the integrity of collateral circulation.[47]

When clinical evidence of cerebral vascular disease is present, the EEG does tend to have focal abnormalities. Yet in a study of asymptomatic, chronic cerebral vascular insufficiency involving the middle cerebral artery, Bruens, Gastaut, and Giove[3] recognized a pattern of paroxysmal regular theta activity, unilateral or bilateral, in the temporal and anterior temporal regions. This showed a marked predominance in the left hemisphere. In most cases, the background rhythm was hardly disturbed. This record was characteristic for aged people with minor disturbances of the middle cerebral artery without serious organic sequelae. Bruens thought that his findings indicated relative ischemia of the sylvian region that might have diagnostic and prognostic implications.

In another study[2] carried out for cerebral localization of infarction and ischemia, there was evidence of unilateral disease in 62 per cent of the patients. EEG abnormalities during the acute phase correlated poorly with the specific site and severity of infarction. In massive infarction, there was diffuse low amplitude delta activity or suppression of electrical activity over the affected hemisphere, whereas high-voltage slow waves seemed to be associated more with localized lesions. Thrombosis of the middle cerebral artery produced diffuse delta activity over the involved hemisphere with theta activity frequently involving the margins of the lesion, though on occasion all activity in the hemisphere might be suppressed (Fig. 7).

In 48 cases of supratentorial occlusive vascular lesions, slow wave foci occurred in 32.[10] Alpha rhythm on the side of the lesion was slowed in the presence of slow wave foci in 50 per cent of the cases. This slowing of the temporoparieto-occipital rhythm was most characteristic at the border of the lesion rather than in the occipital pole as such. There was a preponderance of fast activity in the opposite hemisphere in 28 of the 48 patients, sufficiently marked to be considered as a slightly abnormal sign itself.

Paddison and Ferriss[41] reported a high proportion of abnormal EEG's in patients with cerebral hemisphere infarction secondary to occlusion of the carotid and middle cerebral circulation, in contrast to the frequent occurrence

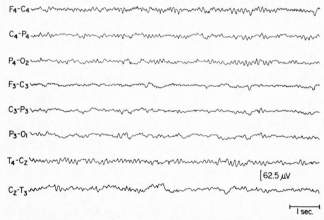

Figure 7. Patient with cerebral infarction due to a left middle cerebral artery obstruction. In the EEG recording there is suppression of background activity and low-voltage slowing.

of normal records in patients with brainstem infarction due to vertebral or basilar artery disease. Five out of six patients with occlusion of the internal carotid or middle cerebral artery had asymmetrically abnormal rhythms.

The cerebral effects of carotid artery disease as manifested electroencephalographically have been further evaluated by Shimizu and Garoutte.[49] Clinical records, EEG's, and carotid arteriograms were studied in 44 aged patients with a clinical diagnosis of "cerebral vascular disease." The EEG was abnormal in 30 (19 focal and 11 diffuse). Twenty-four had unilateral and 5 had bilateral stenosis of the internal carotid artery. When definite EEG focal changes were seen, they were always on the same side as the arterial lesions. On the other hand, unilateral carotid artery abnormalities were associated with EEG abnormalities on the same side in only 10 of 24 cases. Fifteen normal arteriograms were associated with 6 left-sided and 2 right-sided EEG foci. The EEG foci were central and temporal in location, never in the frontal or occipital regions.

Phillips[42] evaluated 40 patients with major and minor syndromes of the basilar-vertebral circulation. Nineteen of the recordings were within normal limits. Phillips pointed out that the EEG is correlated with the disease only in about half the patients. The presence of a normal EEG, however, is evidence that the diencephalic and mesencephalic structures have not suffered severe damage. When the infarction occurs at the pontine level or below, there is no electrographic alteration; when this occurs rostral to the pons, there is generalized bilateral slowing in the electroencephalogram. Among the other abnormalities noted in this series were bitemporal disturbances (activity from 2 to 6 Hz), which were found in 13 of the 21 records.

Birchfield, Wilson, and Heyman[2] reported that in basilar artery thrombosis

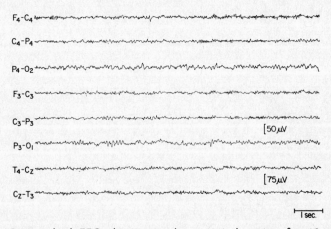

Figure 8. Patient had EEG slowing in the occipital region for 13 years. At autopsy, basilar artery disease was confirmed. There had been no other localizing neurological features during his life.

there is bilateral theta activity in the occipital and posterior temporal regions (Fig. 8). Similarly, Paddison and Ferriss [41] reported that 14 out of 20 patients with vertebral-basilar artery disease had abnormal electroencephalograms characterized by asymmetry of the occipital amplitude and a suppression of alpha.

Correlative studies of cerebral blood flow and the EEG have for the most part indicated a relationship between diminished regional blood flow and slow waves. Ingvar[19] and Magnus, Venderberg, and Vanderdrift[32] were able to demonstrate a significant relationship between the two procedures. There were, however, significant numbers of cases in which there was no correlation. Both authors felt that slow waves were a good indicator of decreased blood flow or metabolism or both. Loeb and Fieschi[28] were less enthusiastic.

TUMORS AND OTHER INTRACRANIAL MASSES

Odom and Friedman[40] have recently called attention to the high incidence of tumors and hematomas in the elderly population. They emphasize the frequent occurrence of intellectual and personality changes as the presenting symptoms. Although these changes can be transitory, they are generally progressive. It is not surprising that the patients are often considered to have the more common forms of dementia and are, as a result, admitted to psychiatric facilities.

Of the 227 patients studied by Odom and Friedman, 69 per cent had intracranial tumors, 21 per cent subdural hematoma, 8 per cent intracerebral hematomas, and another 2 per cent lesions due to epidural hematoma, abscess, and intracerebral cyst. The tumors were gliomas (62 per cent), metastatic (22 per cent), meningiomas (9 per cent), neurinomas (4 per cent), and sarcomas (3 per cent). Eighty-six per cent of the EEG's in these patients were abnormal. The EEG was highly accurate in determining the presence of intracerebral tumor (93 per cent) and subdural hematoma (100 per cent), less accurate in meningioma and in intracerebral hematoma (75 per cent), and even less so in patients with neurinoma (50 per cent).

Brain tumors produce changes in the electroencephalogram that are dependent on two factors.[12] The first is the site of the tumor, for tumors involving the subcortical structures do not produce the same changes that occur with cortical lesions, nor does a temporal lobe tumor affect the EEG in the same way as one in the parietal lobe. The second is the histological and gross anatomical growth characteristics of the lesion since, for example, the EEG changes with an oligodendroglioma are frequently not the same as those that occur with a meningioma.

Gliomas are by far the most common supratentorial neoplasms, invading the brain substance locally and destroying its histological integrity. Epileptic discharges will be more or less common, depending on growth rate. Glioblastomas produce the least epileptic discharge; oligodendrogliomas, the

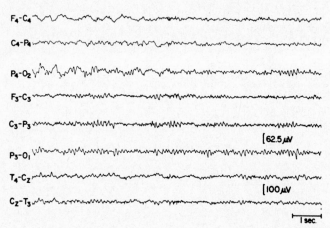

Figure 9. Patient with right parietal lobe tumor. Histopathological diagnosis was mixed glioma. The EEG demonstrates localization of the abnormality to the right central region.

most. Slow wave abnormalities (Fig. 9), on the other hand, are the predominant abnormality with glioblastomas and may be inconspicuous with oligodendrogliomas. Astrocytomas are intermediate; that is, one can expect to see both slowing and epileptic discharge. Neuroblastomas also produce both epileptic discharge and slow waves much like the astrocytoma. Bilateral slow wave abnormalities that arise as a result of subcortical distortion are most likely to occur with rapidly expanding lesions or with those invading subcortical structures. Thus, glioblastomas produce these abnormalities much quicker than oligodendrogliomas.

In contrast to invasive tumors are those that grow as a homogeneous mass within the substance of the brain, not disturbing the histological picture of the surrounding brain except as they distort with the pressure of their growth or result in a foreign body reaction of the brain. In this group, therefore, minimal epileptic discharge is expected, and slowing is predicted to be the predominant change. Such observations correlate well with the studies of Fischer-Williams and associates,[12] Ellingson and Lundy,[8] and Klass and Bickford,[20] who all noted the paucity of epileptic discharge in metastatic tumors. Ellingson and Lundy's excellent summary also emphasized the high frequency of intellectual deficits in patients with metastatic lesions. They made several generalizations that are useful in the diagnosis of dementia: (1) A focal abnormality is highly correlated with a solitary metastasis. (2) Diffuse abnormalities do not correlate with single or multiple metastases unless progression is shown in serial records. (3) A normal record suggests that a metastasis does not exist. (4) Localization of metastases is less accurate than with primary tumors of the brain.

Extrinsic lesions of the brain, such as meningiomas[55] and subdural hematomas,[44,54] produce quite similar findings, suppressing background alpha rhythms in at least one half of the cases. Lateralized and localized slowing is the primary finding in both; epileptic discharges appear in about one half of the patients with meningiomas but are relatively rare in subdural hematomas. Lateralization and localization are accurate in about 86 per cent of the meningiomas, and lateralization is apparent in 75 per cent of patients with subdural hematomas (Fig. 10).

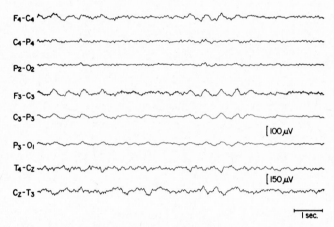

Figure 10. A 79-year-old female who fell, sustaining a head injury. The EEG prior to surgery demonstrated lateralizing slow wave activity over the left frontocentral region. Subsequently, a subdural hematoma was evacuated from the left central region.

CEREBRAL METABOLIC DISORDERS

It is essential to consider briefly chronic metabolic problems that result in changes in the sensorium. Most important from a diagnostic and therapeutic standpoint are the endocrinopathies,[58] in particular myxedema, and pernicious anemia[46, 56] (Fig. 11). Although these entities are most frequently present with psychiatric disturbances of affect, symptoms of delirium and dementia may occur. With either the endocrinopathies or cyanocobalamin deficiency, the EEG may be abnormal. The findings are quite similar in that slowing of the background rhythms in the parieto-occipital region may be the only or earliest finding. Such generalized slowing of the background rhythms occurs in many disorders, such as uremia and hepatic failure, which result in diffuse brain dysfunction. Generalized paroxysmal slowing as well as focal slowing was observed by Walton and his group[56] in a few patients with pernicious anemia.

93

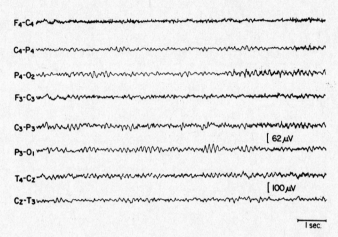

Figure 11. A 55-year-old female with pernicious anemia. This EEG illustrates slowing of the alpha rhythm to 6 to 6½ Hz with a general slowing of the background rhythms. In addition, there is an increase in beta activity in the anterior head regions. The patient had mild sensorial disturbances.

SUMMARY

The EEG in normal aging and in dementia due to a variety of diseases has been described as have the EEG findings in cerebrovascular disease and with intracranial masses. With dementia, the diffuseness of the abnormalities observed has been emphasized, whereas with cerebrovascular disease and with intracranial masses, the focal nature of the changes has been stressed. It is apparent that the EEG can be a significant instrument in the differential diagnosis of dementia. As the test is easily applied, is safe, and can be frequently repeated, it should be considered one of the more useful tools in the clinical examination of patients with dementia.

REFERENCES

1. ABBOTT, J.: *The EEG in Jakob-Creutzfeldt's disease.* Electroenceph. Clin. Neurophysiol. 11:184, 1959.

2. BIRCHFIELD, R. I., WILSON, W. P., AND HEYMAN, A.: *An evaluation of EEG in cerebral infarction and ischemia due to arteriosclerosis.* Neurology 9:859-870, 1959.

3. BRUENS, J. H., GASTAUT, H., AND GIOVE, G.: *EEG study of the signs of chronic vascular insufficiency of the sylvian region in aged people.* Electroenceph. Clin. Neurophysiol. 12:283-295, 1960.

4. BUSSE, E. W., BARNES, R. H., FRIEDMAN, E. L., AND KELTY, E. J.: *Psychological functioning of aged individuals with normal and abnormal electroencephalograms. I. A study of non-hospitalized community volunteers.* J. Nerv. Ment. Dis. 124:135-141, 1956.

5. COBB, W. A.: The normal adult EEG, in Hill, J. D., and Parr, G. (eds.): *Electroencephalography*. The Macmillan Company, New York, 1963, p. 234.

6. DAVIS, P. A.: *The electroencephalogram in old age*. Dis. Nerv. Syst. 2:77, 1941.

7. DAVIS, P. A., AND DAVIS, H.: *The electroencephalograms of psychotic patients*. Amer. J. Psychiat. 95:1007-1025, 1939.

8. ELLINGSON, R. J., AND LUNDY, B. W.: *EEG's in patients suspected of having metastatic lesions of the brain*. Cancer 15:1138-1141, 1953.

9. ENGLAND, A. C., SCHWAB, R. S., AND PETERSON, E.: *The EEG and Parkinson's syndrome*. Electroenceph. Clin. Neurophysiol. 11:723-731, 1959.

10. FARBROT, O.: *EEG study in cases of cerebral vascular accidents*. Electroenceph. Clin. Neurophysiol. 6:678-681, 1954.

11. FISHER, C. M.: *The clinical picture in Creutzfeldt-Jakob disease*. Trans. Am. Neurol. Assn. 85:147-150, 1960.

12. FISCHER-WILLIAMS, M., LAST, S. L., LYBERI, G., AND NORTHFIELD, D. W. C.: *Clinico-EEG study of 128 gliomas and 50 intracranial metastatic tumors*. Brain 85:1-46, 1962.

13. FRIEDLANDER, W. J.: *Electroencephalographic alpha rate in adults as a function of age*. Geriatrics 13:29-31, 1958.

14. GORDON, E. G., AND SIM, M.: *The EEG in pre-senile dementia*. J. Neurol. Neurosurg. Psychiat. 30:285-291, 1967.

15. GOWERS, W. R.: *Heredity in disease of the central nervous system*. Brit. Med. J. 2:1541-1543, 1908.

16. HILL, D.: *Discussion on the electro-encephalogram in organic cerebral disease*. Proc. Roy. Soc. Med. 41:242-248, 1948.

17. HOCH, P., AND KUBIS, J.: *Electroencephalographic studies in organic psychoses*. Amer. J. Psychiat. 98:404-408, 1941.

18. HOEFER, P.F.A.: Discussion of paper by C. M. Fisher.[11]

19. INGVAR, D. H.: *Cerebral metabolism, cerebral blood flow and EEG*. Electroenceph. Clin. Neurophysiol. Suppl. 25:102-106, 1967.

20. KLASS, D. W., AND BICKFORD, R. G.: *The EEG in metastatic tumours of the brain*. Neurology 8:333-337, 1958.

21. KLEIN, R., AND MAYER-GROSS, W.: *The Clinical Examination of Patients with Organic Cerebral Disease*. Cassell and Co., London, 1957.

22. LESSE, S., HOEFER, P. F. A., AND AUSTIN, J. H.: *The electroencephalogram in diffuse encephalopathies*. Arch. Neurol. Psychiat. 79:359-375, 1958.

23 LETEMENDIA, F., AND PAMPIGLIONE, G.: *Clinical and EEG observations in Alzheimer's disease*. J. Neurol. Neurosurg. Psychiat. 21:167-172, 1958.

24. LEVIN, S., AND GREENBLATT, M.: *Electroencephalography in cases with cortical atrophy and ventricular dilation*. Amer. J. Psychiat. 105:220-223, 1948.

25. LIBERSON, W. T.: *Abnormal brain waves and intellectual impairment*. Digest Neurol. Psychiat. 12:234-248, 1944.

26. LIBERSON, W. T., AND SEQUIN, C. A.: *Brain waves and clinical features in arteriosclerotic and senile mental patients.* Psychosom. Med. 1:30-35, 1945.

27. LIDDELL, D. W.: *Investigations of EEG findings in presenile dementia.* J. Neurol. Neurosurg. Psychiat. 21:173-176, 1958.

28. LOEB, C., AND FIESCHI, C.: *EEGs and regional cerebral blood flow in cases of brain infarction.* Electroenceph. Clin. Neurophysiol. Suppl. 25:111-118, 1967.

29. LUCE, R. A., AND ROTHSCHILD, D.: *The correlation of electroencephalographic and clinical observations in psychiatric patients over 65.* J. Gerontol. 8:167-170, 1953.

30. McADAM, W., AND McCLATCHEY, W. T.: *The electroencephalogram in aged patients of a mental hospital.* J. Ment. Sci. 98:711-715, 1952.

31. McADAM, W., AND ROBINSON, R. A.: *Senile intellectual deterioration and the electroencephalogram: A quantitative correlation.* J. Ment. Sci. 102:819-825, 1956.

32. MAGNUS, O., VENDERBERG, D., AND VANDERDRIFT, H. A.: *EEG and cerebral circulation-isotope technique.* Electroenceph. Clin. Neurophysiol. Suppl. 25:107-110, 1967.

33. MAY, W. W.: *Creutzfeldt-Jakob disease.* Acta. Neurol. Scand. 44:1-32, 1968.

34. MULLER, H. F., AND KRAL, V. A.: *The electroencephalogram in advanced senile dementia.* J. Amer. Geriat. Soc. 15:415-426, 1967.

35. MUNDY-CASTLE, A. C., HURST, L. A., BEERSTECHEN, D. M., AND PRINSLOV, T.: *The electroencephalogram in the senile psychoses.* Electroenceph. Clin. Neurophysiol. 6:245-252, 1954.

36. MURPHY, J. T., GLOOR, P., YAMAMOTO, Y. T., AND FEINDEL, W.: *A comparison of electroencephalography and brain scan in supratentorial tumors.* New Eng. J. Med. 276:309-313, 1967.

37. NELSON, J.: *On the origin of diffuse spikes in Jakob-Creutzfeldt's disease.* Electroenceph. Clin. Neurophysiol. 24:395, 1968.

38. OBRIST, W. D.: *The electroencephalogram of normal aged adults.* Electroenceph. Clin. Neurophysiol. 6:235-244, 1954.

39. OBRIST, W. D., AND BUSSE, E. W.: The electroencephalogram in old age, in W. P. Wilson (ed.): *Applications of Electroencephalography in Psychiatry.* Duke University Press, Durham, N. C., 1965, pp. 185-205.

40. ODOM, G. L., AND FRIEDMAN, H.: *Expanding intracranial lesions in geriatric patients.* To be published.

41. PADDISON, R. M., AND FERRIS, G. S.: *EEG in cerebral vascular disease.* Electroenceph. Clin. Neurophysiol. 13:99-110, 1961.

42. PHILLIPS, B. M.: *Temporal lobe changes associated with the syndromes of basilar-vertebral insufficiency: An EEG study.* Brit. Med. J. 2:1104-1107, 1964.

43. POLLOCK, M., AND HORNABROOK, R. W.: *The prevalence, natural history and dementia of Parkinson's disease.* Brain 89:429-448, 1966.

44. PUECH, P., BOUNES, G. C., AND LUQUET, P.: *Chronic, latent, subdural hematoma. Neuropsychiatric signs and EEG studies.* Ann. Med. Psychiat. 11:158, 1947.

45. RUBIN, M. A.: *Electroencephalographic localization of atrophy in the cerebral cortex of man.* Proc. Soc. Exp. Biol. 40:153-154, 1939.

46. SAMSON, D. C., SWISHER, S. N., CHRISTIAN, R. M., AND ENGEL, G. L.: *Cerebral metabolic disturbance and delirium in pernicious anemia.* Arch. Int. Med. 90:4-14, 1952.

47. SCHWAB, R. S.: EEG studies and their significance in cerebral vascular disease, in Wright, I. S. (ed.) : *Cerebral Vascular Diseases.* Grune & Stratton, New York, 1955, pp. 123-132.

48. SCHWAB, R. S., AND COBB, S.: *Simultaneous electromyograms and EEGs in paralysis agitans.* J. Neurophysiol. 2:36-41, 1939.

49. SHIMIZU, M., AND GAROUTTE, B.: *EEG and carotid arteriography in elderly patients.* Electroenceph. Clin. Neurophysiol. 24:394, 1968.

50. SHORT, M. J., MUSELLA, L., AND WILSON, W. P.: *Correlation of affect and EEG in senile psychoses.* J. Gerontol. 23:324-327, 1968.

51. SILVERMAN, A. J., BUSSE, E. W., AND BARNES, R. H.: *Studies in the process of aging: Electroencephalographic findings in 400 elderly subjects.* Electroenceph. Clin. Neurophysiol. 7:67-74, 1955.

52. TASKER, R. R., AND SCOTT, J. W.: *The prognostic value of the EEG in thalamotomy for parkinsonism.* Electroenceph. Clin. Neurophysiol. 21: 620, 1966.

53. TROWBRIDGE, E. J., JR., AND FINLEY, K. H.: *The electroencephalogram and pneumoencephalogram in non-focal neurological disorders.* Amer. J. Roentgenol. Rad. Ther. 47:699-702, 1942.

54. TURRELL, R. C., LEVY, L. L., AND ROSEMAN, E.: *The value of EEG in selected cases of subdural hematomas.* J. Neurosurg. 13:449-454, 1956.

55. WAJSBORT, J., LAVY, S., SAHAR, A., AND CARMON, A.: *The value of EEG in the diagnosis and localization of meningioma.* Confin. Neurol. 28:375-384, 1966.

56. WALTON, J. N., KILOH, L. G., OSSELTON, J. W., AND FARRALL, J.: *The electroencephalogram in pernicious anaemia and subacute combined degeneration of the cord.* Electroenceph. Clin. Neurophysiol. 6:45-64, 1954.

57. WEINER, H., AND SCHUSTER, D. B.: *The electroencephalogram in dementia —some preliminary observations and correlations.* Electroenceph. Clin. Neurophysiol. 8:479-488, 1956.

58. WILSON, W. P.: The EEG in endocrine disorders, in Wilson, W. P. (ed.) : *Applications of Electroencephalography in Psychiatry.* Duke University Press, Durham, N. C., 1965, pp. 102-122.

Chapter 6

Radiological Procedures in the Diagnosis of Dementia

William F. Meacham, M.D., and
A. Byron Young, M.D.

The proper investigation of the cause of dementia requires radiographic studies whenever the cause has not been discovered by the usual careful history and physical examination.

The use of the special diagnostic procedures discussed here has two primary objectives: (1) to demonstrate focal lesions (as neoplasm, subdural hematoma, and localized atrophy) causing dementia; (2) to demonstrate diffuse lesions ("normal pressure hydrocephalus," diffuse cerebral atrophy, as examples) causing dementia. The diagnostic methods employed are not mutually exclusive, and the approach varies with the individual patient. If the clinical features lead the physician to suspect a focal lesion, he will most often proceed directly in an attempt to demonstrate its presence. If the clinical features lead the physician to suspect a diffuse lesion, he will usually perform several relatively atraumatic diagnostic procedures that are known to demonstrate a large proportion of focal lesions presenting without focal signs. Failing in the demonstration of a focal lesion, he may then proceed to tests specifically designed to demonstrate diffuse lesions.

SKULL X-RAY EXAMINATIONS

The initial evaluation should include routine x-ray examinations of the skull. The standard projections consist of stereoscopic lateral views, a posterior-anterior view, and a half-axial or Towne's projection. The clues to possible disease on the routine skull films include, among others, such significant findings as a shifted or displaced calcified pineal body, intracranial calcifications associated with neoplastic disease, pressure erosion of the sella and convexity, spreading of the sutures, and abnormal bony vascular channels. The discovery of any of these abnormalities is sufficiently important to require further clarification of the problem with appropriate additional studies. The fact that skull x-ray findings are normal must not (contrary to popular thought) be considered reassuring, since most diseases of the brain occur without producing detectable radiographic changes in the skull.

STUDIES FOR DEMONSTRATION OF FOCAL LESIONS

Brain Scanning

The use of radioactive isotopes has revolutionized certain aspects of diagnostic neurology. The affinity of certain lesions for these isotopes in far greater proportions than normal brain tissue or the surrounding integuments has resulted in quick, painless, and often accurate localization of neoplasms, hematomas, vascular malformations, abscesses, infarcts, and cysts. The most commonly used isotopes are compounds of mercury or technetium, although others are receiving clinical and experimental study. The counting and recording devices employed in "brain scanning" are cumbersome and expensive marvels of technical ingenuity. Now combined with computerized methods of recording, very sophisticated scans can be made with increasing accuracy. Studies of this sort are not considered harmful and, thus far, seem free of risk to the patient.

While these methods are not infallible and a normal scan does not rule out a mass lesion, the percentage of reliability is high and is increasing with experience and with technical improvement. In a recent review, Maynard and Janeway[10] reported the accuracy of brain scanning for neoplasm to vary between 65 and 95 per cent in different published series, being 81.5 per cent in their own laboratory. This compared in their own series with an accuracy of neoplasm localization of 45 per cent by skull films, 92.3 per cent by angiography, and 93.9 per cent by air studies. Brain scanning is also frequently positive in the localization of cerebral infarction, subdural hematoma, arteriovenous malformation, brain abscess, and lesions of the skull and scalp. There is no abnormality on brain-scan studies in degenerative diseases, and the test is of value primarily in detecting the silent or suspected mass lesion.

Angiography

Cerebral angiography ranks second only to pneumoencephalography and ventriculography in importance in neurological diagnostic procedures. De-

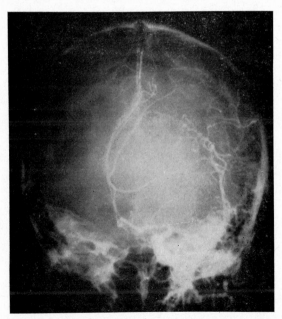

Figure 1. Carotid arteriogram. There is a massive displacement of the anterior cerebral artery past the midline. This is diagnostic of a mass lesion in the frontal lobe.

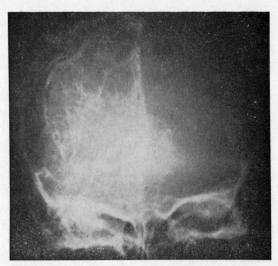

Figure 2. Carotid arteriogram. Late arterial phase showing a large avascular space between the surface of the hemisphere and the inner table of the skull. A characteristic finding in chronic subdural hematoma.

scribed first by Moniz in 1927, it was not widely accepted until relatively nonirritating contrast materials were developed. Angiography is particularly useful in the detection of mass lesions of the cerebral hemispheres. It also can yield specific information concerning the relative vascularity of tumors, the source of the major blood supply, the location of the principal cerebral arteries, and can suggest the actual histological type of neoplasm (meningiomas and glioblastomas, for example) in a respectable number of instances (Fig. 1). This study also is effectively employed in the diagnosis of vascular occlusive disease, cerebral atrophy, intracranial hematomas (Fig. 2), arterial and venous aneurysms, and arteriovenous malformations. Careful study of the various phases of the angiographic picture can disclose subtle shifts in the midline structures, denote ventricular size, and give valuable clinical information regarding the efficiency of the circle of Willis and other perfusion peculiarities of the cerebral circulation.

An additional advantage from the use of cerebral angiography is the tolerance shown by patients who might be harmed by the disturbances in their intracranial pressure effected by air-contrast studies, thus obviating the necessity for immediate craniotomy. Cerebral angiography currently carries a low morbidity, and fatalities related to the procedure are a rarity. The principal disadvantages to the procedure are those that apply to all diagnostic studies of this sort, i.e., diagnostic accuracy that depends on the distortion and displacement of normal structures or the development of abnormal circulation may fail to reveal the early lesion or those situated in certain "blind" areas of the intracranial compartment.

Air Studies

The use of air, or other gases, as an opacifying medium for the subarachnoid spaces and the ventricular system has been continuous and widespread since it was first employed by Dandy in 1918. By using total cerebrospinal fluid–air exchange, total or global pneumography is employed to demonstrate the entire ventricular system and the subarachnoid spaces. The use of smaller amounts of air (fractional pneumography), which is the common practice today, demonstrates virtually all of the intracranial cavities, but requires repeated position changes to allow the gas to enter each topographical area on the basis of posture. This achieves the advantage of eliminating superimposition of air shadows and also lessens the morbidity associated with all methods of spinal air injection. Headache, nausea, and meningismus are almost invariable accompaniments of pneumography, but these symptoms are transient and usually subside by the end of 24 to 48 hours. The inhalation of 95 per cent oxygen may reduce the severity and duration of the headache, presumably by hastening the absorption of nitrogen across the subarachnoid-vascular barrier.

Visualization of the subarachnoid spaces and the ventricles makes it possible to diagnose many intracranial disorders. Distortion and displacement of the ventricles may signify a mass lesion or the effects of cicatricial contraction on ventricular walls; dilatation of the ventricles may indicate an obstructive process or compensatory enlargement due to focal or generalized cerebral cortical atrophy or hypoplasia; typical deformities may be disclosed, indicating the presence of congenital abnormalities such as agenesis of the corpus callosum, porencephaly, cerebral aplasia, aqueductal atresia, the Arnold-Chiari malformation, and others. The patient with dementia due to a degenerative process may reveal striking enlargement of the ventricles and pooling of air in the sulci and subarachnoid spaces overlying atrophic cerebral or cerebellar hemispheres (see below).

When adequate visualization of the intracranial fluid compartments cannot be obtained as a result of failure of the air to enter the ventricular system because of obstruction or technical difficulties, air may be injected directly into the ventricles by transcortical ventricular puncture (Fig. 3). This method of air injection (ventriculography) is usually employed in those cases exhibiting degrees of frank intracranial hypertension, under which circumstance there may be prohibitive risk associated with pneumography via the spinal route. This requires, except in infants, a surgical opening of the skull (burr openings) to allow needle passage into the ventricular cavity. This method offers an additional advantage in allowing a cortical or brain biopsy to be taken during the procedure, outweighing to some extent the disadvantage of the shaven head and the imposed surgical procedure. Combined ventricular and spinal air injections may occasionally be required to produce adequate visualization of all the structures to which

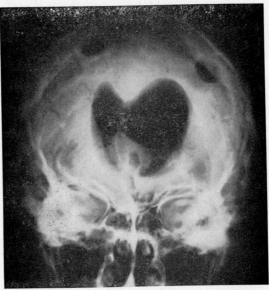

Figure 3. Ventriculogram. Direct injection of air into the ventricles. Excessive enlargement of the ventricles is present. The opaque, spherical, colloid cyst may be seen, which has obstructed the foramina of Monro.

clinical interest is directed. Pneumography remains one of the most important and helpful diagnostic tools employed in clinical neurology. Its use requires a special degree of expertise in its performance as well as in the radiographic interpretation; it should never be performed casually or when not specifically indicated.

STUDIES FOR DEMONSTRATION OF DIFFUSE LESIONS

RISA Scanning

An important clinical discovery in recent years has been the description of the peculiar syndrome known as "low pressure hydrocephalus," "normal pressure hydrocephalus," or "occult hydrocephalus."[1] Following trauma, infections, hemorrhage, or for unknown reasons, the development of progressive hydrocephalus without the signs of increased intracranial pressure has occurred and results in a clinical picture of disorientation, confusion, and obtundity, often associated with signs of long-tract dysfunction and cerebellar dysfunction. A basic fault in the circulation-absorption pattern of the cerebrospinal fluid develops so that there is free communication between the ventricular system and the spinal subarachnoid space, but the flow of the fluid into the basilar cisternae and over the convexities of the hemispheres to the areas of absorption at the arachnoidal villi is absent, or seriously impaired. This produces insidious and progressive ventricular dilatation at the expense of the cerebral parenchyma. This loss equilibrates with the increased ventricular volume, so that the pressure is compensated.

Appreciation of this condition and its treatment has resulted in the reversal of catastrophic intellectual impairment in many victims of this disorder in recent years. By the utilization of a special technique of isotope scanning as introduced by Di Chiro[5] in 1964, the condition may be diagnosed with certainty. When radioactive iodinated serum albumin (RISA) is injected by lumbar puncture into the subarachnoid space, it moves upward, first into the cisterna magna, thence over the surfaces of the cerebral hemispheres where it is concentrated along the site of the superior longitudinal sinus where it is absorbed into the blood. In the normal individual, the radioactivity is detected in the basal cisterns within about an hour after

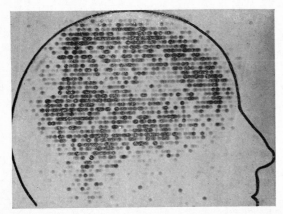

Figure 4. RISA scan. Demonstrates the "normal" pattern of radioactive concentrations in the basilar cisternae, convexity subarachnoid spaces, and at the sagittal sinus area. This is the pattern seen in "hydrocephalus ex vacuo."

injection and over the cerebral convexities near the superior longitudinal sinus after 12 to 24 hours (Fig. 4), after which radioactivity rapidly fades. Little or no radioactivity appears in the ventricles in the normal subject. The study is well tolerated and can be combined with lumbar puncture for diagnostic study of the spinal fluid if desired. Repeat scanning of the brain area is done at 24, 48, and, if necessary, 72 hours after injection before a final diagnosis is made on the basis of the scan information.

In general, RISA scans are considered to be abnormal (Fig. 5): (1) when there is reflux of radioactive material in the ventricles at 24 hours after injection; (2) when little or no radioactivity appears over the cerebral convexities following lumbar intrathecal injection; or (3) when the process of movement upward, collection over the cerebral convexities, and absorption into the bloodstream is appreciably slowed.[7]

105

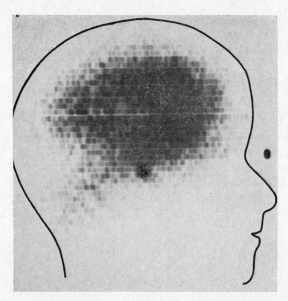

Figure 5. RISA scan. Reveals concentration of the radioactive material in the excessively dilated ventricles. The material was injected into the lumbar subarachnoid space 24 hours previously. This is the typical "scan" picture of occult or low pressure hydrocephalus.

Several studies have been published in recent years detailing the normal and abnormal findings in RISA scanning.[2, 5, 7-9] In one recent study[7] of 130 patients with dementia or with dilated ventricles (as demonstrated by air studies), abnormal RISA scans were observed in 25 patients. Ventricular reflux without isotopic activity over the convexities was observed in 17 patients while delayed flow was seen in 8. When dementia was present alone, the occurrence of positive RISA scans was uncommon, but the incidence increased with dementia plus long tract signs or cerebellar signs.

When the diagnosis is confirmed, ventriculoatrial shunting has resulted in recovery or improvement in many instances. With additional experience and increasing technological improvement, such methods may shed additional light on abnormalities of cerebrospinal fluid circulation and absorption.

Angiography

Cerebral contrast angiography is not usually performed with a view to the demonstration of diffuse cerebral lesions, though signs suggesting diffuse disease may be a helpful by-product of such studies performed in search of a focal defect. Increased sweep of the anterior cerebral arteries has long been an accepted sign of enlarged lateral ventricles. Heinz, Davis, and Karp[7] have recently called attention to the "stretching of the pericallosal artery over the corpus callosum" in patients with obstructive hydrocephalus, contrasting this with the pattern seen in cerebral atrophy with ventricular enlargement where the "normal undulations" of the artery are retained even though the sweep is increased. Cerebral angiographic studies may indicate cerebral atrophy also by revealing an avascular subdural "gap" as well as demonstrating ventricular enlargement by a changed configuration of the thalamostriate veins that outline the inferolateral walls of the lateral ventricles.

Air Studies

The use of air to opacify the subarachnoid spaces and ventricular system (usually by lumbar intrathecal injection) has as its objective the demonstration of two prime diffuse lesions: (1) diffuse atrophy of brain substance, and (2) "normal pressure hydrocephalus."

DIFFUSE CEREBRAL ATROPHY. Diffuse atrophy of brain substance is demonstrated pneumoencephalographically by a widening and deepening of the cerebral sulci (often with "puddles" of air seen overlying the atrophic gyri) and by a diffuse enlargement of the cerebral ventricles (Fig. 6). The experienced clinician usually evaluates the air encephalogram on a subjective basis, making the assessment of normality or abnormality on the basis of long experience in evaluating the size and configuration of cerebral sulci

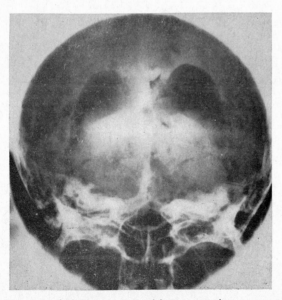

Figure 6. Pneumoencephalogram. In addition to the symmetrically dilated ventricles there are puddles of air over the surface, indicating enlargement of the sulci and atrophy of the parenchyma.

and ventricles. Numerous efforts have been made to make the measurement of cerebral atrophy more precise.

Although some authors have thought it impossible to establish exact radiological criteria for the diagnosis of widening of cerebral sulci, others have accepted 3 mm. as the maximal normal width for cerebral sulci as demonstrated encephalographically.[11,13] Using this criterion, Nielsen and co-workers[11] have studied a large series of patients with pneumoencephalograms. They observed that though cortical atrophy is frequently most apparent in the frontal areas, wide sulci in one region are usually accompanied by widening of sulci in other regions as well. In their study, sulcal widening was rare below the age of 40 years though ventricular enlargement might be striking at early ages. They thus found cortical atrophy, to a greater extent than ventricular enlargement, to be a product of the process of aging. They also found a fairly close correlation between the degree of intellectual deterioration and the degree of cortical atrophy.

Numerous attempts have also been made to quantitate ventricular enlargement. Since rounding and blunting of the lateral ventricular angles is often an early sign of ventricular enlargement, Taveras and Wood[13] devised a measurement based on this portion. Others have measured width of the lateral ventricles,[4, 12] height of the lateral ventricles,[12] diagonal diameter of the lateral ventricles,[6] width of the floor of the lateral ventricles,[3] and the upper angle of the lateral ventricle.[6] Most thoroughly studied has been the width of the bodies of the lateral ventricles, or the "ventricular span" as it has been called by Burhenne and Davies.[4] Their figure of 45 mm. as the upper limit of the maximal spread of the bodies of the lateral ventricles appears most apposite. The width of the third ventricle has also been widely studied, and an upper limit of 7 mm. is most generally accepted.[12, 13] There is "an obvious correlation"[12] between the width of the third ventricle and the size of the lateral ventricles, though the correlation is far from perfect. There is also some correlation between ventricular size and the age of the patient.[12]

Both ventricular enlargement and widening of the cortical sulci are correlated with the severity of intellectual impairment,[11,12] though the correlation for the latter is better than for the former.[11] Despite a relationship between ventricular enlargement and sulcal widening, one cannot predict atrophy in one region from the presence of atrophy in the other.[11]

NORMAL PRESSURE HYDROCEPHALUS. In this condition, the pneumoencephalographic picture is characteristic. After lumbar intrathecal injection, air readily fills the ventricular system, which always reveals rather distinct dilatation of the lateral and third ventricles, although the cerebral aqueduct and the fourth ventricle may be normal in size. The convexity subarachnoid spaces fail to fill with air, although in some instances the basilar cisterns and the sylvian fissure and adjacent sulci may contain some air (Fig. 7). When no air appears outside the ventricles, there is little

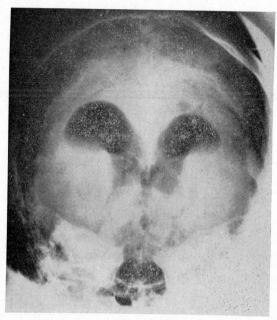

Figure 7. Pneumoencephalogram. The lateral ventricles are moderately enlarged and symmetrical, and there is a paucity of air over the surfaces of the hemisphere. Such a pattern is compatible with occult hydrocephalus.

question as to diagnosis. When a small amount of air is seen in the basilar cisterns and above the tentorium, however, definite diagnosis is more difficult and other clues are needed. Dilatation of the fourth ventricle and the aqueduct is often striking in normal pressure hydrocephalus,[1,7] while it usually is insignificant in patients with cerebral atrophic disease. When pneumoencephalographic signs of normal pressure hydrocephalus are equivocal, RISA scanning may be of particular value.[7]

REFERENCES

1. ADAMS, R. D., FISHER, C. M., HAKIM, S., OJEMANN, R. G., AND SWEET, W. H.: *Symptomatic occult hydrocephalus with "normal" cerebrospinal pressure.* New Eng. J. Med. 273:117, 1965.

2. BANNISTER, R., GILFORD, E., AND KOCEN, R.: *Isotope encephalography in the diagnosis of dementia due to communicating hydrocephalus.* Lancet 2:1014, 1967.

3. BULL, J. W. D.: *The volume of the cerebral ventricles.* Neurology 11:1, 1961.

4. BURHENNE, H. J., AND DAVIES, H.: *The ventricular span in cerebral pneumography.* Amer. J. Roentgenol. 90:1176, 1963.

5. DI CHIRO, G.: *New radiographic and isotopic procedures in neurological diagnosis.* J.A.M.A. 188:524, 1964.

6. GOSLIN, R. H.: *The association of dementia with radiologically demonstrated cerebral atrophy.* J. Neurol. Neurosurg. Psychiat. 18:129, 1955.

7. HEINZ, E. R., DAVIS, D. O., AND KARP, H. R.: *Abnormal isotope cisternography in symptomatic occult hydrocephalus.* Radiology 95:109, 1970.

8. KILGORE, B. B., DAVIS, D. O., AND POTCHEN, E. J.: *Abnormal cerebrospinal fluid dynamics as studied by isotope subarachnoid scintigraphy.* Acta Radiol. (diag.) 9:626, 1969.

9. LIN, J. P., GOODKIN, R., TONG, E. C. K., EPSTEIN, F. J., AND VINCIGUERRA, E.: *Radioiodinated serum albumin (RISA) cisternography in the diagnosis of incisural block and occult hydrocephalus.* Radiology 90:36, 1968.

10. MAYNARD, C. D., AND JANEWAY, R.: Radioisotope studies in neurodiagnosis, in Toole, J. F. (ed.): *Special Techniques for Neurologic Diagnosis.* F. A. Davis Co., Philadelphia, 1969, pp. 71-91.

11. NIELSEN, R., PETERSEN, O., THYGESEN, P., AND WILLANGER, R.: *Encephalographic cortical atrophy.* Acta Radiol. (diag.) 4:437, 1966.

12. NIELSEN, R., PETERSEN, O., THYGESEN, P., AND WILLANGER, R.: *Encephalographic ventricular atrophy.* Acta Radiol. (diag.) 4:240, 1966.

13. TAVERAS, J. M., AND WOOD, E. H.: *Diagnostic Neuroradiology.* The Williams & Wilkins Co., Baltimore, 1964.

Chapter 7

Studies in the Pathology of Dementia

Richard M. Torack, M.D.

The classification of the group of neurological disorders collectively labeled *dementia* is based on certain clinical, chemical, and morphological findings indicative of cortical neuronal dysfunction since specific etiological agents have not been identified in most of these conditions. Any attempt to achieve a purely morphological classification of dementia is difficult because the structural changes in cortical neurons are neither consistent nor specific. For example, the differentiation between senile dementia and Alzheimer's disease rests on the age of the patient and not on the presence of senile plaques or neurofibrillary tangles, which are regularly found in both conditions. Therefore it is not surprising that the existing divisions are frequently arbitrary and controversial.[42]

A particular form of dementia secondary to arteriosclerotic vascular disease is generally acknowledged and consists of either multiple cortical infarcts or laminar necrosis due to the resultant cortical ischemia

A group of the dementias is also recognized with a chronic clinical course (more than 2 years) in which the cortex contains a distinctive neuronal alteration consisting of senile plaques, neurofibrillary tangles, granulovacuolar degeneration, and large argyrophilic inclusion bodies (i.e., Alzheimer's disease, Pick's disease, senile dementia, and Mariana dementia).

Another dementing syndrome is recognized with a subacute clinical course (2 months to 2 years) in which neuronal cell loss is unaccompanied by characteristic changes in neurons (e.g., Jakob-Creutzfeldt disease).

Finally, there are numerous examples of chronic dementia in which neuronal cell loss is unaccompanied by distinctive changes in neurons or in blood vessels. These may exist as a separate entity or as part of a syndrome such as Huntington's chorea or Wilson's disease. In these conditions pathological features other than the character of the neuronal degeneration may allow a precise disease diagnosis on pathological examination.

From this discussion, one can readily appreciate that while neurons malfunction or die in all these conditions, particular structural abnormalities of neurons occur only in the groups usually called *presenile* and *senile dementia*. Furthermore, since no specific neuronal changes occur in the other dementing syndromes, it is apparent that neurons can die rapidly or slowly without having a distinctive structural abnormality. Accordingly, two immediate problems are posed for a discussion of the morphological correlates in dementia: first, to evaluate how the distinctive changes in neurons are related to neuron death; second, to find a significant cellular abnormality that could explain neuronal degeneration in the absence of a distinctive morphological change.

This chapter is devoted largely to an examination of neuronal morphology in both subacute and chronic varieties of dementia, particularly to the morphological changes revealed by electron microscopy. No attempt is made here to review the gross and light microscopic pathology of the many disease states

112

that result in the clinical condition termed dementia. Such would provide merely a replication of the excellent review of McMenemey,[40] to which the reader is referred. This essay constitutes rather a critical review of recent studies on the ultrastructure of brain as they throw light on the many disorders appearing clinically as dementia.

DISTINCTIVE NEURONAL MORPHOLOGY IN CHRONIC DEMENTIA

These cortical morphological changes include neurofibrillary tangles, senile plaques, granulovacuolar degeneration, and argentophilic inclusion bodies. While these alterations are not limited to cortical neurons in chronic dementia, their frequent occurrence in this disease strongly implies a close relationship to the evolution of neuronal degeneration. Specifically they are characteristic of senile dementia, Alzheimer's disease, Pick's disease, and the dementia found in the Mariana Islands as part of the dementia-parkinsonism—amyotrophic lateral sclerosis complex. All can be identified occasionally in brains (particularly in the temporal lobe[67]) of elderly people not clinically recognized as demented. In this sense, the concept of "premature aging" of neurons has been justified. However, this viewpoint does not help us understand neuronal degeneration whether it occurs at age 35 or at age 85. Accordingly, a critical evaluation of these changes in terms of altered cell biology is indicated.

Neurofibrillary Tangles

This neuronal alteration was first described by Alzheimer[2] in the disease bearing his name. Similar structures are prominent in neurons in senile dementia, Pick's disease, the dementia complex on Guam,[29] and postencephalitic parkinsonism.[24] Recent ultrastructural findings have confirmed that the tangles are irregular masses of neurofilaments,[33,37,64] and a most important advance concerning these cytoplasmic organelles has resulted from their experimental production by aluminum salts[34,66] and particularly by colchicine and other mitotic spindle inhibitors.[74,76] Similar cytoplasmic structures in normal cells appear to be composed of contractile proteins.[51,61] These neurofilaments have been shown to be important in the saltatory movements occurring within many types if not all cells.[17,50] In neurons, axoplasmic flow[36] as well as the movements of specific formed organelles such as neurosecretory granules[53] and lysosomes[41] appears to be mediated by these neurofilaments. Microtubules and neurofilaments are believed by some to be interchangeable, and colchicine, periwinkle alkaloids, podophyllin, and griseofulvin appear to alter this interaction.[76] In neurons and in other cells, aggregates of filaments (e.g., neurofibrillary tangles) and microtubular crystals are produced by these compounds,[3,54,74] and an interference with the aforementioned cytoplasmic movements accrues. Interestingly, although an obvious defect in the assembly of these protein structures is present, neither the biochemical assay of cortical biopsy material of Alzheimer's disease[63] nor of individual neurons treated with vincristine[12] reveals any diminution in the uptake of labeled protein. However, abnormal neurofilaments affecting axoplasmic flow could result in a deprivation of essential proteins to the axon, which might explain neuronal dysfunction under these circumstances. Impaired intracellular digestion as a result of lysosomal dysfunction could lead to an accumulation of toxic metabolites and cell death. The elucidation of this cytoplasmic abnormality represents a most significant advance in our understanding of neuronal disease in dementia. Since many substances are capable of inducing this change, however, the etiological agent could be endogenous or exogenous and remains unidentified at this time.

Senile Plaques

These complex structures originally were described by Blocq and Marinesco[5] in 1892 and have been considered to be the result of neuronal degeneration,[6] glial degeneration,[5] or a degeneration of the intercellular ground substance.[72] Recent electron microscopic studies of senile plaques[37,39,65] have not clarified this controversy, for the plaques were found to contain cellular and extracellular material, possibly related to all three sources (i.e., neurons, glia, and intercellular ground substance). The center appears to be composed of extracellular material, histochemically and morphologically characteristic of amyloid.[11,25] Surrounding this irregular core is an intertwined array of cell processes, including those of neurons with many neurofibrils, of glial cells, and of mesodermal cells, presumably the origin of the amyloid. Altered synapses have been observed in these plaques.[22] Histochemical and biochemical studies have revealed other interesting enzymatic and chemical characteristics of senile plaques.[18,63] Which component of this cellular and extracellular array is the "vis movendi"?

Probably the distinctive feature of the plaque is the presence of amyloid. The most recent experimental data concerning amyloid deposition indicate that certain proteins (e.g., casein) can stimulate its deposition in tissues. This tissue response appears to result from the presence of the protein itself, plus an amyloid-enhancing factor (AEF), produced by reticulocytes of the spleen in response to such a protein. The protein and the AEF pass by the blood to tissue histiocytes, which then produce the extracellular fibrillar material we call amyloid.[32] Occasionally in systemic amyloidosis, plaque formation in the brain can occur, although the more common finding is vascular amyloidosis.[26] The relationship of plaque formation to neuronal dysfunction is obscure, and if neuronal processes were not involved in "senile plaques," no correlation would appear warranted. Certainly the frequent association of senile plaques with neurofibrillary tangles is equally perplexing. As amyloid deposition appears to be related to a circulating factor and the tangles can be produced by exogenous materials, an abnormality of vascular permeability is needed to allow such an agent or agents to enter the brain and produce these changes.

Granulovacuolar Change

Alzheimer[1] again deserves recognition as the first to describe this neuronal abnormality, which consists of small vacuoles in the cytoplasm or at the base of dendrites in degenerating neurons, each vacuole containing at its center a small granule. Granulovacuolar changes are most prevalent in the temporal lobe, particularly in the pyramidal cells of Ammon's horn, which has led some investigators to believe the change to be specific for this type of cell.[57] It has been considered by some to be a step in the production of neurofibrillary tangles.[44] However, such granules have not been observed in the experimental production of neurofibrillary tangles,[75] and their etiology or significance remains obscure. Hirano and associates[28] have collected electron micrographs of these bodies in autopsy tissue from cases of Parkinson-dementia on Guam and have confirmed a membrane-limited vacuole with a dense center. The origin of these bodies, whether from lysosomes, phagosomes, or endoplasmic reticulum, was not revealed. The material in the membrane-bound vacuole may represent either an abnormal substance or a normal material that is not degraded. Hirano and his group[28] have noted an association of neurons containing granulovacuolar change with other neurons containing crystals, but a relationship to impaired autodigestion (which may exist from blocked microtubule formation) remains entirely speculative.

Pick's Inclusions

Although the clinical entity was first described by Pick[48] this specific histological change was characterized initially by Alzheimer.[1] These inclusions can sometimes be extremely prominent, especially in neurons of the temporal lobe. Recently Schochet, Lampert, and Lindenberg[55] have demonstrated the ultrastructure of these bodies in autopsy material. These electron micrographs suggest that the inclusions are not membrane bound and that they possess a composition of granular and filamentous material. The granules are said to be morphologically similar to ribosomes, while the filaments are about 200Å in diameter. This suggests a relationship between polysomes and neurofilaments, but no convincing evidence that polysomes manufacture these contractile proteins is available at this time.

In summary, in the neurons of patients with dementia, neurofibrillary tangles are the only distinctive change about which there is some understanding regarding cause and evolution. The presence of such degenerative forms in senile dementia, Alzheimer's disease, and Pick's disease is a strong argument that a factor affecting contractile cytoplasmic protein is acting in all these conditions. There is experimental evidence that several compounds are capable of experimentally inducing such an effect. The variable clinical course, the different topographic distribution of brain involvement, and the occurrence of other distinctive degenerative forms in this group of dementias could conceivably indicate that specific agents having specific neuronal predilection cause these syndromes. However, until such data are obtained, the distinction between these entities must remain empirical.

NEURONAL DEGENERATION IN DEMENTIA NOT CHARACTERIZED BY DISTINCTIVE MORPHOLOGICAL ALTERATION OF NEURONS

This rather heterogenous group of dementias has been subdivided according to the presence or absence of vascular disease, the rapidity of the dementing process, or an association with a more generalized disorder. However, in each case, the surviving neurons exhibit an altered morphology like that found in a wide variety of diseases ranging from anoxia to the Werdnig-Hoffmann syndrome, in which no dementing syndrome has been described. Morphological changes such as increased satellitosis, chromatolysis, and sclerosis certainly evoke no concept of a specific degenerative process or a particular etiological agent. The dementia occurring in the presence of vascular disease suggests an ischemic basis for the cell death. Since this is primarily an extraneuronal disease, perhaps the occurrence of similar nonspecific neuronal change in the other disorders is a hint that we should not look for the primary change in neurons.

Among the dementias not characterized by specific neuronal structural change or the presence of vascular disease, the rapidity of the degenerative process has been most widely used as a distinguishing characteristic. In this way, a category of subacute dementia has been established and generally identified by the eponym Creutzfeldt-Jakob disease or Jakob-Creutzfeldt disease. A lack of structural uniformity has existed from the first descriptions of this group, for Creutzfeldt's case (1920) [9] did not have the severe vacuolization and gliosis characteristic of two of Jakob's cases (1921) .[31] Various attempts, beginning with Heidenhain,[27] have been made to achieve greater specificity through the identification of more uniform and specific subgroups. However, these efforts have not gained unanimous approval. Probably the most successful classification is that more recently popularized by Nevin and associates,[46] who collected a group of patients having similar clinical and pathological abnormalities, which they called *subacute spongiform encephalopathy*. These workers appreciated Heidenhain's observations that his cases and some of Jakob's[31] had severe vacuolization of the cortex. Actually more significant differences also exist between the subacute spongiform encephalopathy group and those examples subsumed under the Jakob-Creutzfeldt eponym. Those cases described first by Heidenhain and later collected by Nevin and associates[45] had severe neuronal loss and a distinct reactive gliosis with maximal involvement in the occipital lobes, but the other brains showed minimal neuronal loss, prominent satellitosis of neurons, and little gliosis with maximum involvement outside the occipital lobes. Appropriately more recently, *subacute spongiform degeneration* has become the accepted name for the group collected by Nevin and his group,[46] while the other dementias have been termed *classic Jakob-Creutzfeldt disease*.

Less widely appreciated is a group of cases in which prominent striatal-cerebellar degeneration occurs in addition to cortical involvement.[16, 56] The histological findings in these cases include the extensive neuronal loss and marked reactive gliosis but not the marked cystic change previously noted by Heidenhain and Nevin. It follows that these brains are also different from Creutzfeldt's case and those described by Jakob without the cystic change. A total of ten cases of this type was summarized by Brownell and Oppenheimer,[8] and Nevin, Barnard, and McMenemy[45] have reported another. The present problem is whether these are sufficiently distinct from the Heidenhain-Nevin variety to merit a separate categorization. The prominent cerebellar involvement and the lack of severe spongiosis are arguments for separation, yet the reactive gliosis and neuronal loss are similar to the Heidenhain-Nevin cases. The most convincing argument for regarding all these patients as belonging to one group is the patient reported by Gibbs and colleagues.[21] In this patient, brain biopsy revealed rather typical changes of spongiform encephalopathy, but at autopsy several months later the changes were consistent with those described by Brownell and Oppenheimer.[8]

Very significantly, in 1968 Gibbs and co-workers[21] reported the transmission of Creutzfeldt-Jakob's disease from the patient just described to a monkey, suggesting the cause of the disorder to be a slow virus. The following year, Gibbs and Gajdusek[20] reported successful transmission from man to monkey in six of eight patients suffering from spongiform encephalopathy. More recently, Vernon, Fuccillo, and Hamilton[70] and Vernon and associates[71] have reported the observation of virus-like particles by electron microscopy in two patients with spongiform encephalopathy. Thus strong evidence now supports the viral etiology of subacute spongiform encephalopathy, a variety of Jakob-Creutzfeldt disease. The only other significant etiological factor so far proposed is a hereditary metabolic defect, which is suggested by the rare incidence of familial subacute dementia.[43]

The classification of the remaining dementias, usually having a chronic clinical course, comes perilously close to complete chaos. In Huntington's chorea the hereditary factor must be significant; in Wilson's disease abnormal copper metabolism is implicated; in hepatic failure, ammonia may or may not be a significant factor. Other chronic dementing syndromes not identified with specific diseases are completely ignored, quickly forgotten, or labeled *atypical*. These problems cannot be resolved at this time, but recent investigations have begun to clarify our understanding of these dementias.

Subacute Dementia

As mentioned earlier, three categories in this group (the "classic" Jakob-Creutzfeldt group, the Heidenhain-Nevin group called subacute spongiform encephalopathy, and the Brownell-Oppenheimer group) have come to be tentatively recognized by neuropathologists. Unfortunately, especially in the past, many studies of these subgroups have been related only to the more general category and designated only as Jakob-Creutzfeldt disease. Therefore, the results of these studies can only be retrospectively identified with one of the more particular variants. All of these conditions are associated with some degree of neuronal cell loss as observed in light-microscopic preparations with no distinctive morphology of the surviving neurons. In subacute spongiform degeneration, Gonatas, Terry, and Weiss[23] have characterized the fine structure of neurons as having numerous lipofuscin bodies essentially identical to those occurring in aging neurons.[52] Friede and DeJong[19] characterized these neurons histochemically as having low oxidative enzymatic activity and regarded the disease of neurons as one of enzymatic failure. Biochemical studies have revealed a reduction of gangliosides and cholinesterase,[49,62] but these can be explained on the basis of neuronal cell loss. No particular chemical change, such as the accumulation of acid mucopolysaccharide in Alzheimer's disease, is noted in subacute dementia. Suzuki and Chen[62] and Korey, Katzman, and Orloff[35] have noted an increase in glycolipids in the gray matter, but this has been related to the prominent gliosis found in all of the variants of this syndrome. The nature of the severe spongy degenerative change has been identi-

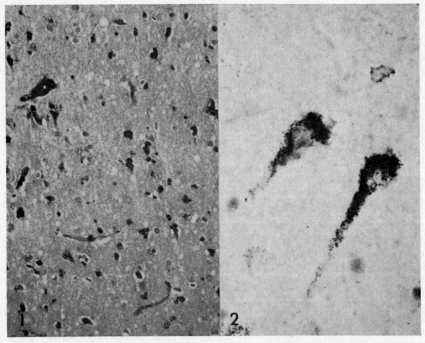

Figure 1. A photomicrograph of cortex from a biopsy in subacute dementia in which a moderate neuronal loss is visible. PAS stain × 40.

Figure 2. A photomicrograph of two cortical neurons in tissue, which are reacted to demonstrate acid phosphatase activity. A granular reaction product is visible filling the perikaryon and the proximal axons. × 400.

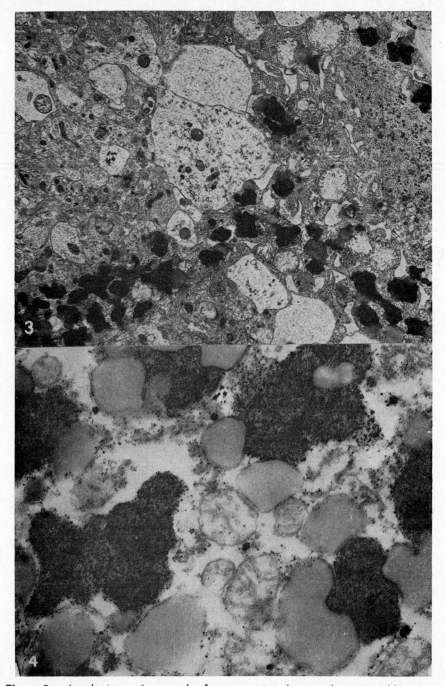

Figure 3. An electron micrograph of a neuron in subacute dementia. Numerous lipofuscin bodies fill the perikaryon and proximal axon. $\times$ 10,000.

Figure 4. This tissue has been incubated in the Gomori medium to demonstrate acid phosphatase activity at pH 5.0. The final product is localized to the dense component of these neuronal dense bodies. $\times$ 30,000.

fied by Gonatas, Terry and Weiss,[23] and it consists of a massive dilatation of astrocytes, a finding confirmed by Sluga and Seitelberger.[58] Apart from these dilated astrocytes seen in subacute spongiform degeneration, however, no distinctive ultrastructural or chemical correlate has been related to any of the subgroups identified by light microscopic and clinical findings.

I have had an opportunity to obtain for study a biopsy from each of the three variants of subacute dementia. Two of these cases have been reported elsewhere.[69] The third, an example of cortico-striatal-cerebellar degeneration, has been more recently obtained and confirmed by autopsy after the patient's illness of 6 months' duration. Unfortunately, no chemical studies have been performed on this latter tissue. In each of these patients, light microscopic examination of the biopsy reveals a mild to severe loss of neurons in the cortex with no other significant neuronal change (Fig. 1). In the case of subacute spongiform degeneration there was a marked cystic change in the cortex in the biopsy and in the autopsy tissue. Both the subacute spongiform degeneration and the cortico-striatal-cerebellar degeneration have a significant degree of reactive gliosis either in the biopsy, in the autopsy, or in both. Acid phosphatase activity is increased in cortical neurons of the case of classical Jakob-Creutzfeldt disease and of the subacute spongiform degeneration (Fig. 2).

Electron microscopic examination of these biopsies has revealed the neurons of all variants to be essentially similar (Fig. 3). They all contain numerous dense bodies, closely resembling lipofuscin as previously described by Gonatas, Terry, and Weiss.[23] These bodies fill the perikaryon and the proximal axon. In the two cases that have been investigated for enzyme activity, these bodies are also the site of the acid phosphatase activity where the reaction product is limited to the dense component of these bodies (Fig. 4). Between these lipofuscin-like bodies, little rough endoplasmic reticulum

Table I. A tabulation of recent pathological data pertinent to the classification of subacute dementia

	Classical Jakob-Creutzfeldt Disease	Subacute Spongiform Degeneration	Cortico-Striatal-Cerebellar Degeneration
Neurons	±Cell loss	++Cell loss	++Cell loss
	++Dense bodies	++Dense bodies	++Dense bodies
	++AcPO₄ase	++AcPO₄ase	Not performed
Glia	±Reactive	++Dilated	±Dilated
		++Reactive	++Reactive
Blood Vessels	++Basement membrane thickening	Normal	Normal

(Nissl material) is visible; however, since cortical neurons vary so much in their content of Nissl material, a definite reduction in rough endoplasmic reticulum is very difficult to evaluate. The fine structure in the case of sub-acute spongiform degeneration reveals numerous greatly dilated astrocytes as others have described. The case of classical Jakob-Creutzfeldt disease has a previously undescribed finding, namely, capillaries with greatly thickened basement membranes.[67] A summary of the significant data resulting from these studies in subacute dementia is presented in Table 1.

Chronic Dementia

The existence of dementing syndromes lasting more than 2 years and having none of the morphological stigmata of presenile dementia has always been recognized; however, these cases are so heterogeneous that their existence as a distinct group of diseases appears questionable. The presence of a variable clinical presentation coupled with the light microscopic finding of only neuronal loss and variable gliosis fails to evoke any concept of specific abnormality. Little recent ultrastructural or chemical assay of such tissue is available.

Cortical biopsies of two patients having dementia for more than 3 years have been studied with histochemical, biochemical, and ultrastructural techniques at The New York Hospital. One of these has been previously reported.[68] These two cases of chronic dementia were characterized clinically by periodic exacerbations, followed by some improvement but never to the functional level that existed prior to the worsening symptoms. Light microscopic examination of the cortex revealed a mild to moderate loss of neurons, no significant increase in acid phosphatase activity, and no other histological change. Electron microscopic studies revealed most of the neurons to be normal; however, perhaps 20 per cent of the cortical neurons contained prominent compound dense bodies (Fig. 5 and 6). These organelles have a dense granular component similar to a lipofuscin body, and they are characterized by containing an abnormally large amount of pale homogeneous material, also found in lipofuscin bodies. The acid phosphatase activity is present only in the dense granular component. Furthermore, occasionally the pale homogeneous component is found within a saccular extension of the endoplasmic reticulum (Fig. 6). Since this material resembles unsaturated lipid that accumulates in the endoplasmic reticulum in fatty livers,[14,59] sections of cortex were digested with pancreatic lipase, phospholipase C, trypsin, and chymotrypsin to identify the chemical nature of the material. Only pancreatic lipase removed the pale homogeneous component (Fig. 7). While the other enzymes affected the osmiophilia of the two components, neither of these was removed by their action. The pale material has been tentatively identified as triglyceride in this way.[4]

One of these biopsies from a patient with chronic dementia was performed shortly following an exacerbation of mental deterioration at a time when

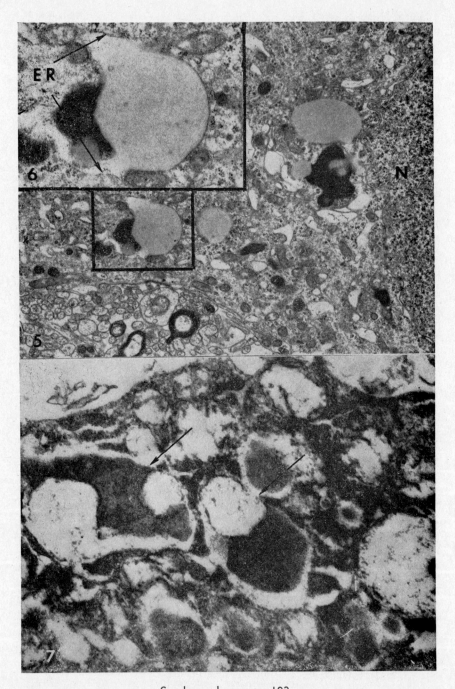

See legend on page 123.

some improvement in mental status had been noted. In this biopsy some neurons are seen in which the nuclear membrane contains numerous nuclear pores, present throughout the nuclear circumference, in addition to the abnormal dense bodies (Fig. 8). Within some of these pores, granular material having approximately the same density as ribosomes can be identified (Fig. 9). In both biopsies a mild increase of fibrous astrocytes is visible. No specific vascular change is present in either case.

SIGNIFICANCE OF LYSOSOMES IN DEGENERATING NEURONS IN DEMENTIA

The evaluation of the importance of lipofuscin and lipid materials in neuronal degeneration obviously must be done with great caution. Lipofuscin bodies are generally believed to be a form of lysosome.[52] The presence of acid phosphatase in these bodies is consistent with this concept. The evolution of these dense bodies from the Golgi apparatus and from the endoplasmic reticulum is diagramed in Figure 10. Lysosomes have been shown to occur in normal and abnormal cells as a cellular mechanism for the degradation of endogenous or exogenous material.[10,30,47] Their appearance in injured cells is considered to be a cellular reaction in an attempt to destroy either an injuring agent, injured part of the cell, or cell organelles that may not be necessary to maintain life under adverse circumstances. Therefore, they must be considered a response to cell injury and not a prime indicator of specific cell damage.

In the neurons from the cases of subacute dementia, the great increase in lipofuscin bodies correlates well with the severity of the disease process. In other words, the bodies reflect serious neuronal injury, the nature of which remains obscure. Previously the glial alteration in subacute spongiform degeneration and the peculiar thickening of vascular basement membranes in the other case described above were considered more specific changes.[69] The possibility of these changes affecting neuronal nutrition has been discussed, but

←————————————————————————————

Figure 5. The ultrastructure of an abnormal neuron (N) in a case of chronic dementia reveals dense bodies in which the predominant component is a pale homogeneous substance. ✕ 10,000.

Figure 6. An enlargement of the dense body in the insert of Figure 5. The pale homogeneous component is delimited by membranes continuous with the endoplasmic reticulum (ER). ✕ 22,000.

Figure 7. This is a frozen section of tissue from the same biopsy represented in Figures 5 and 6, which has been digested in an aqueous solution containing 20 mg. pancreatic lipase (activity at least 100 units/mg.) at pH 8.0 for 2 hours prior to preparation for electron microscopy. At least two dense bodies are visible (arrows) and the pale homogeneous substance appears to be completely removed. ✕ 22,000.

123

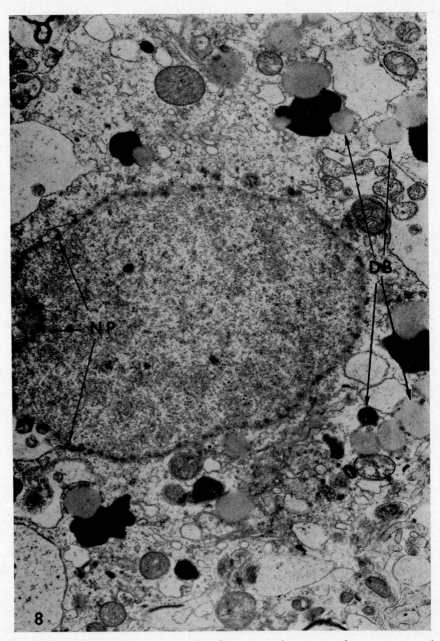

Figure 8. An electron micrograph of a cortical neuron of a patient with chronic dementia who has manifested some clinical improvement. The nuclear membrane contains numerous nuclear pores (NP). Dense bodies (DB) with a prominent pale homogeneous component are visible in the cytoplasm. $\times$ 12,000.

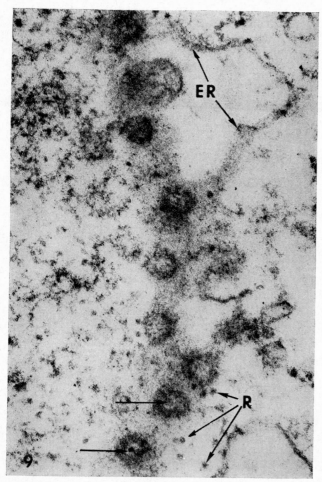

Figure 9. A higher magnification of the nuclear pores reveals some pores to contain granular material (arrows) having an electron density similar to ribosomes (R). Membranes of endoplasmic reticulum (ER) are visible. × 70,000.

there is no evidence to indicate their etiological basis. The demonstration of virus-like particles[70,71] in these tissues and the transmission of spongiform encephalopathy[20] and of cortico-striatal-cerebellar degeneration[21] to the monkey argue for an infectious etiology.

The neuronal changes in the chronic dementias are even more intriguing. Lipofuscin bodies normally contain a small amount of pale homogeneous material, but the presence of an increased amount of this substance in a lipofuscin body is abnormal. Hirano[28] noted similar bodies in the Mariana cases. This material, which appears to be a triglyceride on the basis of the digestion studies, seems to originate from the endoplasmic reticulum. The endoplasmic

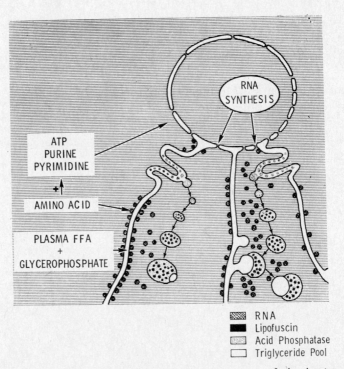

RNA
Lipofuscin
Acid Phosphatase
Triglyceride Pool

Figure 10. The left half of this diagram depicts some of the basic structural pathways for protein and lipid synthesis of normal cells. (Modified after Farber, 1966.[13]) Schematically it depicts the origin of a membrane-bound lipofuscin body (also containing acid phosphatase) from a folded network of smooth membranes, termed the Golgi complex. On the right-hand portion of the drawing, structural changes are shown that could lead to a formation of the odd lipofuscin bodies found in neurons in dementia. Of particular interest is the incorporation of a large lipid component derived from the endoplasmic reticulum.

reticulum in liver cells has been shown to have a triglyceride pool that is used to synthesize lipoproteins, conjugated lipids, cholesterol, and cholesterol esters.[14] When one or more of these synthetic processes are inhibited, triglyceride accumulates.[14,59] Inhibition of lipoprotein synthesis apparently results in fatty liver in this way.[14]

Some indication of abnormal neuronal protein synthesis is revealed by the presence of many nuclear pores in the case biopsied during a recuperative phase. The presence of numerous nuclear pores is generally considered to indicate increased transfer of nucleoprotein from nucleus to cytoplasm[15,60,73] where the nucleoprotein is used to synthesize various cellular proteins. Increased nuclear pores can be observed in a variety of cells, but in neurons they have been seen best in regenerating neurons on about the tenth day following axon section.[38] At this time, increased protein synthesis is apparent chemically in these neurons.[7] An antecedent derangement of protein synthesis is implied if increased protein synthesis is found in the biopsied neurons. In this regard, the chromatolysis commonly seen in these biopsies may achieve greater significance, since this is believed to indicate decreased cytoplasmic RNA. As previously mentioned and as noted in Figure 10, such abnormal protein synthesis would explain the increased lipid of the compound dense body. The importance of these findings of abnormal protein synthesis is that they appear to indicate a new pattern of neuronal degeneration that at least in some cases appears reversible. Since protein synthesis can be altered in many ways, no indication of a specific etiological agent is presented by these studies. The ultimate separation of the dementias in these categories must await the recognition of the etiological agent.

SUMMARY

The existing classification of human dementia has been noted to be both arbitrary and confusing. These diseases appear to be validly distinguished by the presence or absence of arteriosclerosis, the presence or absence of distinctive neuronal structural changes, and the rapidity of the dementing process.

In the group containing distinctive neuronal changes, the presence of neurofibrillary degeneration appears to be most significant. The importance of this alteration accrues from its widespread occurrence and from its experimental production by a variety of agents, particularly those classified as spindle inhibitors. These latter compounds appear to block the normal formation of neurofilaments and microtubules, which have been shown to be important in intracellular transport. By interfering with axon transport and intracellular digestion, neuronal dysfunction or death can occur. Since many substances can produce these effects, specific classification within this group of dementias must await the identification of the etiological agent.

The remaining categories of dementia have no distinctive neuronal structural change, and a serious doubt arises whether the etiological agent is acting primarily upon the neurons. In some, vascular or glial abnormalities appear somewhat specific, and these have been considered to be the primary disease, with secondary involvement of neurons. Apart from increased acid phosphatase activity, no light microscopic distinction is noted in these neurons. Ultrastructural studies have revealed an increased number of dense bodies, in which acid phosphatase activity is located. Abnormally large amounts of simple lipid, which in one case was shown to arise from the endoplasmic reticulum, can be seen in some of these dense bodies. This finding, coupled with the occurrence of numerous nuclear pores, suggests that some inhibition of protein metabolism is occurring in these cells. These findings are generally believed to be secondary cellular responses, however, and, although they appear to indicate a pattern of neuronal degeneration, absolute categorization awaits an identification of specific causative agents. An infectious agent, specifically a slow virus, must be considered the most likely possibility at this time. Although these morphological and chemical changes may not indicate specific etiological agents, they do provide more insight into the way neurons are altered and offer additional criteria for the ultimate separation of these entities.

REFERENCES

1. ALZHEIMER, A.: *Ueber eigenartige Krankheitsfaelle des spaetern Alters.* Z. ges. Neurol. Psychiat. 4:356, 1911.

2. ALZHEIMER, A.: *Ueber eine eigenartige Erkrankung der Hirnrinde.* Cbl. Nervenheilk. Psychiat. 18:177-179, 1907.

3. BENSCH, K. G., AND MALAWISTA, S. E.: *Microtubular crystals in mammalian cells.* J. Cell Biol. 40:95-107, 1969.

4. BIER, M.: Lipases, in Colowick, S. P., and Kaplan, N. O. (eds.) : *Methods in Enzymology.* Academic Press, New York, 1955, vol. 1, pp. 627-642.

5. BLOCQ, P., AND MARINESCO, G.: *Sur les lésions et la pathologie de l'épilepsie dite essentiale.* Sem. Med. Paris 12:445-446, 1892.

6. BONFIGLIO, E.: *Di speciali reperti in un caso di probabile sifilide cerebrale.* Riv. Sper. Freniat. 34:196, 1908.

7. BRATTGARD, S. O., HYDEN, H., AND SJÖSTRAND, J.: *Incorporation of orotic acid-C^{14}, and lysine C^{14} in regenerating single nerve cells.* Nature 182: 801-802, 1958.

8. BROWNELL, B., AND OPPENHEIMER, D. R.: *An ataxic form of subacute presenile polioencephalopathy (Creutzfeldt-Jakob disease).* J. Neurol. Neurosurg. Psychiat. 28:350-361, 1965.

9. CREUTZFELDT, H. G.: *Ueber eine eigenartige herdfoermige Erkrankung des Zentralnervensystems.* Z. ges. Neurol. Psychiat. 56:1-18, 1920.

10. DEDUVE, C., AND WATTIAUX, R.: *Functions of lysosomes.* Ann. Rev. Physiol. 28:435-492, 1966.

11. DIVRY, P.: *De la nature de l'altération fibrillaire d'Alzheimer.* J. Belg. Neurol. Psychiat. 34:197-201, 1934.

12. EMBREE, L. J., HAMBERGER, A., AND SJÖSTRAND, J.: *Quantitative cytochemical studies and histochemistry in experimental neurofibrillary degeneration.* J. Neuropath. Exp. Neurol. 26:427-436, 1967.

13. FARBER, E.: *On the pathogenesis of fatty livers.* Gastroenterology 50:137-141, 1966.

14. FARBER, E., SHULL, K. H., VILLA TREVINA, S., LOMBARDI, B., AND THOMAS, M.: *The biochemical pathology of acute hepatic adenosinetriphosphate deficiency.* Nature 203:34-40, 1964.

15. FELDHERR, C. M.: *The nuclear annuli as pathways for nucleocytoplasmic exchanges.* J. Cell Biol. 14:65-72, 1962.

16. FOLEY, J. M., AND DENNY-BROWN, D.: *Subacute progressive encephalopathy with bulbar myoclonus.* J. Neuropath. Exp. Neurol. 16:133-136, 1957.

17. FREED, J. J.: *Microtubules and saltatory movements of cytoplasmic elements in cultured cells.* J. Cell Biol. 27:29A, 1965.

18. FRIEDE, R. L.: *Enzyme histochemical studies of senile plaques.* J. Neuropath. Exp. Neurol. 24:477-491, 1965.

19. FRIEDE, R. L., AND DEJONG, R. N.: *Neuronal enzymatic failure in Creutzfeldt-Jakob disease. A familial study.* Arch. Neurol. 10:181-195, 1964.

20. GIBBS, C. J., JR., AND GADJUSEK, D. C.: *Infection as the etiology of spongiform encephalopathy (Creutzfeldt-Jakob disease).* Science 165:1023-1025, 1969.

21. GIBBS, C. J., JR., GADJUSEK, D. C., ASHER, D. M., ALPERS, M. P., BECK, E., DANIEL, P. M., AND MATTHEWS, W. B.: *Creutzfeldt-Jakob disease (spongiform encephalopathy): Transmission to the chimpanzee.* Science 161:388-389, 1968.

22. GONATAS, N. K., ANDERSON, W., AND EVANGELISTA, I.: *The contribution of altered synapses in the senile plaque. An electron microscopic study in Alzheimer's dementia.* J. Neuropath. Exp. Neurol. 26:25-39, 1967.

23. GONATAS, N. K., TERRY, R. D., AND WEISS, M.: *Electron microscopic study in two cases of Jakob-Creutzfeldt disease.* J. Neuropath. Exp. Neurol. 24:579-598, 1965.

24. GREENFIELD, J. G., AND BOSANQUET, F. D.: *The brain stem lesions in parkinsonism.* J. Neurol. Neurosurg. Psychiat. 16:213-226, 1953.

25. GUEFT, B., AND GHIDONI, J. J.: *The site of formation and ultrastructure of amyloid.* Amer. J. Path. 43:837-854, 1963.

26. HABERLAND, C.: *Primary systemic amyloidosis. Cerebral involvement and senile plaque formation.* J. Neuropath. Exp. Neurol. 23:135-150, 1964.

27. HEIDENHAIN, A.: *Klinische und anatomische Unterschungen ueber eine eigenartige organische Erkrankung des Zentralnervensystems in Praesenium.* Z. ges. Neurol. Psychiat. 118:49-114, 1928.

28. HIRANO, A., DEMBITZER, H. M., KURLAND, L. T., AND ZIMMERMAN, H. M.: *The fine structure of some intraganglionic alterations. Neurofibrillary tangles, granulo-vacuolar bodies and "rod-like" structures as seen in Guam amyotrophic lateral sclerosis and parkinsonism-dementia complex.* J. Neuropath. Exp. Neurol. 27:167-182, 1968.

29. HIRANO, A., MALAMUD, N., ELIZAN, T. S., AND KURLAND, L. T.: *Amyotrophic lateral sclerosis and Parkinson-dementia complex on Guam.* Arch. Neurol. 15:35-51, 1966.

30. HOLTZMAN, E., NAVIKOFF, A. B., AND VILLAVERDE, H.: *Lysosomes and GERL in normal and chromatolytic neurons of the rat ganglion nodosum.* J. Cell Biol. 33:419-435, 1967.

31. JAKOB, A.: *Ueber eigenartige Erkrankungen des Zentralnervensystem mit bemerkenswerten anatomischen Befunden.* Z. ges. Neurol. Psychiat. 64:147-228, 1921.

32. JANIGAN, D. T.: *Pathogenetic mechanisms in protein induced amyloidosis.* Amer. J. Path. 55:379-394, 1969.

33. KIDD, M.: *Alzheimer's disease—an electron microscopical study.* Brain 87:307-320, 1964.

34. KLATZO, I., WISNIEWSKI, H., AND STREICHER, E.: *Experimental production of neurofibrillary degeneration. I. Light microscopic observations.* J. Neuropath. Exp. Neurol. 24:187-210, 1965.

35. KOREY, S. R., KATZMAN, R., AND ORLOFF, J.: *A case of Jakob-Creutzfeldt disease. 2. Analysis of some constituents of the brain of a patient with Jakob-Creutzfeldt disease.* J. Neuropath. Exp. Neurol. 20:95-104, 1961.

36. KREUTZBERG, G. W.: *Histochemical demonstration of a colchicine-induced blockage of enzyme transport in axons of peripheral nerves.* Proc. Int. Cong. Histochem. and Cytochem. Springer-Verlag, New York, 1968, pp. 133-134.

37. KRIGMAN, M. R., FELDMAN, R. G., AND BENSCH, K.: *Alzheimer's presenile dementia. A histochemical and electron microscopic study.* Lab. Invest. 14:381-396, 1965.

38. LAMPERT, P. W. Personal communication.

39. LUSE, S. A., AND SMITH, K. R.: *The ultrastructure of senile plaques.* Amer. J. Path. 44:553-563, 1964.

40. McMENEMEY, W. H.: The dementias and progressive diseases of the basal ganglia, in Blackwood, W., McMenemy, W. H., Meyer, A., Norman, R. M., and Russell, D. S. (eds.) : *Greenfield's Neuropathology,* ed. 2, The Williams & Wilkins Co., Baltimore, 1963.

41. MALAWISTA, S. E.: *Colchicine: A common mechanism for its anti-inflammatory and anti-mitotic effects.* Arthritis Rheum. 11:191-197, 1968.

42. MARGOLIS, C.: *Senile cerebral disease. A critical survey of traditional concepts based upon observations with newer techniques.* Lab. Invest. 8:335-370, 1959.

43. MAY, W. W., ITABASHI, H. H., AND DEJONG, R. N.: *Creutzfeldt-Jakob disease. II. Clinical, pathologic and genetic study of a family.* Arch. Neurol. 19:137-149, 1968.

44. MOREL, F., AND WILDI, E.: *Clinice pathologique générale et cellulaire des altérations seniles et preseniles du cerveau.* Proc. 1st. Int. Cong. Neuropath. (Rome) 2:347, 1952.

45. NEVIN, S., BARNARD, R. O., AND McMENEMEY, W. H.: *Different types of Creutzfeldt-Jakob disease.* Acta Neuropath. (Suppl. III) 9:7-13, 1967.

46. NEVIN, S., McMENEMEY, W. H., BEHRUMAN, S., AND JONES, D. P.: *Subacute spongiform encephalopathy—a subacute form of encephalopathy attributable to vascular dysfunction (spongiform cerebral atrophy).* Brain 83:519-564, 1960.

47. NOVIKOFF, A. B.: Lysosomes in nerve cells, in Hyden, H. (ed.) : *The Neuron.* Elsevier Publishing Co., Amsterdam, Netherlands, 319-366, 1967.

48. PICK, A.: *Ueber einen weiteren Symptomenkomplex.* Mschr. Psychiat. Neurol. 19:97-108, 1906.

49. POPE, A., HESS, H. H., AND LEWIN, E.: Studies on the microchemical pathology of human cerebral cortex, in Cohen, M. M., and Snider, R. S. (eds.): *Morphological and Biochemical Correlates of Neural Activity.* Harper & Row, Publishers, New York, 1964, pp. 98-111.

50. PORTER, K. R.: Cytoplasmic microtubules and their function, in Wolstenholme, G. E. W., and O'Connor, M. (eds.): *Principles of Biomolecular Organization* (Ciba Foundation Symposium). Little, Brown and Company, Boston, 1966, pp. 308-356.

51. RENAUD, F. L., ROWE, A. J., AND GIBBONS, I. R.: *Some properties of the protein forming the outer fibers of cilia.* J. Cell Biol. 36:79-90, 1968.

52. SAMORAJSKI, T., ORDY, J. M., AND KEEFE, J. R.: *The fine structure of lipofuscin age pigment in the nervous system of aged mice.* J. Cell Biol. 26:779-795, 1965.

53. SCHMITT, F. O.: *The molecular biology of neuronal fibrous proteins.* Neurosci. Res. Prog. Bull. 6:119-144, 1968.

54. SCHOCHET, S. S., JR., LAMPERT, P. W., AND EARLE, K. M.: *Neuronal changes induced by intrathecal vincristine sulfate.* J. Neuropath. Exp. Neurol. 27:645-658, 1968.

55. SCHOCHET, S. S., JR., LAMPERT, P. W., AND LINDENBERG, R.: *Fine structure of the Pick and Hirano bodies in a case of Pick's disease.* Acta Neuropath. 11:330-337, 1968.

56. SILBERMAN, J., CRAVIOTO, H., AND FEIGIN, I.: *Cortico-striatal degeneration of the Creutzfeldt-Jakob type.* J. Neuropath. Exp. Neurol. 20:105-118, 1961.

57. SIMCHOWICZ, T.: *Histologische Studien ueber die Senildemenz.* Nissl-Alzheimer Arbeiten 3:268, 1911.

58. SLUGA, E., AND SEITELBERGER, F.: *Beitrag zur spongioesen Encephalopathie.* Acta Neuropath. (Suppl. III) 9:60-72, 1967.

59. SMUCKLER, J., ISERI, O. A., AND BENDITT, E. P.: *An intracellular defect in protein synthesis induced by carbon tetracholoride.* J. Exp. Med. 116:55-71, 1962.

60. STEVENS, B. J., AND SWIFT, H. R.: *NA transport from nucleous to cytoplasm in chronomilus salivary gland.* J. Cell Biol. 31:55-78, 1966.

61. STEVENS, R. E., ROWE, A. J., AND GIBBONS, I. R.: *Guanine nucleotide associated with protein of the outer fibers of flagella and cilia.* Science 156:1606-1608, 1967.

62. SUZUKI, K., AND CHEN, G.: *Chemical studies on Jakob-Creutzfeldt disease.* J. Neuropath. Exp. Neurol. 25:396-408, 1966.

63. SUZUKI, K., KATZMAN, R., AND KOREY, S. R.: *Chemical studies on Alzheimer's disease.* J. Neuropath. Exp. Neurol. 24:211-224, 1965.

64. TERRY, R. D.: *The fine structure of neurofibrillary tangles in Alzheimer's disease.* J. Neuropath. Exp. Neurol. 22:629-642, 1963.

65. TERRY, R. D., GONATAS, N. K., AND WEISS, M.: *Ultrastructural studies in Alzheimer's presenile dementia.* Amer. J. Path. 44:269-297, 1964.

66. TERRY, R. D., AND PENA, C.: *Experimental production of neurofibrillary degeneration. II. Electron microscopy, phosphatase histochemistry and electron probe analysis.* J. Neuropath. Exp. Neurol. 24:200-210, 1965.

67. TOMLINSON, B. E., BLESSED, G., AND ROTH, M.: *Observations on the brains of non-demented old people.* J. Neurol. Sci. 7:331-356, 1968.

68. TORACK, R. M.: *Ultrastructural and histochemical studies in a case of progressive dementia and its relationship to protein metabolism.* Amer. J. Path. 49:77-97, 1966.

69. TORACK, R. M.: *Ultrastructural and histochemical studies of cortical biopsies in subacute dementia.* Acta Neuropath. 13:43-55, 1969.

70. VERNON, M. L.:, FUCCILLO, D. A., AND HAMILTON, R.: *Jakob-Creutzfeldt disease: Virus-like particles in two brain biopsies.* Fed. Proc. 29:286, 1970.

71. VERNON, M. L., HORTA-BARBOSA, L., FUCCILLO, D. A., SEVER, J. L., BARINGER, J. R., AND BIRNBAUM, G.: *Virus-like particles and nucleoprotein-type filaments in brain tissue from two patients with Creutzfeldt-Jakob disease.* Lancet 1:964-966, 1970.

72. VON BRAUNMUEHL, A.: *Neue Gesichtspunkte zum Problem der senilen Plaques.* Z. ges. Neurol. Psychiat. 133:391-411, 1931.

73. WIENER, J., SPIRO, D., AND LOWENSTEIN, W. R.: *Ultrastructure and permeability of nuclear membranes.* J. Cell Biol. 27:107-117, 1965.

74. WISNIEWSKI, H., KARCEZEWSKI, W., AND WISNIEWSKA, K.: *Experimental colchicine encephalopathy. I. Induction of neurofibrillary degeneration.* Lab. Invest. 17:577-587, 1967.

75. WISNIEWSKI, H., NARKIEWICZ, O., AND WISNIEWSKA, K.: *Topography and dynamics of neurofibrillar degeneration in aluminum encephalopathy.* Acta Neuropath. 9:127-133, 1967.

76. WISNIEWSKI, H., SHELANSKI, M. L., AND TERRY, R. D.: *Effects of mitotic spindle inhibitors on neurotubules and neurofilaments in anterior horn cells.* J. Cell Biol. 38:224-229, 1968.

Chapter 8

Biochemical Dysfunction and Dementia*

Stanley H. Appel, M.D., and
Barry W. Festoff, M.D.

* This work has been supported by the Robert McManus Memorial Grant No. 558-B-3 from the National Multiple Sclerosis Society, and Grant No. NB-07872 from the National Institutes of Health, United States Public Health Service.

Previous chapters have defined the range of mental dysfunction and intellectual deterioration associated with the term *dementia*. It is usually applied to a diffuse deterioration in mental function, primarily in thought and memory, and secondarily in feeling and conduct. Dementia is not due to a single cause, but may be the result of inflammatory, vascular, toxic, neoplastic, traumatic, malnutritional, infectious, or degenerative processes.

Chapter 10 details the many diseases that may present with dementia. A most significant point is that the diverse causes of dementia preclude any specific biochemical event as the sole cause. Alterations in vitamin intake (thiamine, niacin, B_{12}, or folic acid), hormones, and electrolyte ions are known to be associated with dementia; yet such substances are involved in a wide range of biochemical reactions, and no single rate-limiting reaction can be applied to all.

The main emphasis of the present chapter will be on the biochemical approaches to the primary dementias, i.e., those in which dementia is the only or dominant symptomatology. If a biochemical cause can be discovered, any specific primary dementia will become secondary to a particular protein, carbohydrate, lipid, or nucleic acid deficiency. In addition, the particular biochemical changes may be secondary to a specific toxic or infectious process. A recent case in point is the demonstration of "slow virus" in biopsy material from a patient with Jakob-Creutzfeldt disease.[28] If such studies are confirmed in this and other dementias, the resulting biochemical changes to be described may themselves be secondary to viral disease.

Since dementia usually is associated with diffuse cerebral dysfunction, the critical element underlying the biochemistry of dementia may be to understand the way in which particular disease processes interfere with normal neuronal and glial function and the way in which the altered neurons participate in communal responses. Are the clinical symptoms of specific dementia expressions of a single metabolic defect, more than one metabolic derangement, or simply vague manifestations of a rate-limiting process in brain function such as communication between cells? Two distinct approaches can be applied to this analysis. The first is to assume that a given metabolic process has been impaired in a diffuse fashion. This approach has been employed in an attempt to understand inborn errors of metabolism and their devastating systemic and cerebral effects. Widespread impairment of energy metabolism; amino acid transport; protein, nucleic acid, lipid or carbohydrate metabolism could cause diffuse dysfunction. Such effects have been accordingly implicated as the biochemical lesion in entities like phenylketonuria and branched-chain amino-aciduria.

Diffuse dysfunction has also been attributed to alterations in cerebral blood flow. Most significant are the observations that the reduction in cerebral blood flow and metabolism in organic dementia are correlated with the severity of mental impairment.[43, 48, 58] Associated with the decreased blood flow Skinhoj[57] demonstrated increased pH in cisternal fluid in patients with severe organic dementia. Sokoloff[58] proposed that tissue anoxia resulting from circulatory deficit is an etiological factor in the reduced cerebral oxygen uptake of such patients. His data suggested that reduced blood flow was secondary to arteriosclerotic disease and, in turn, led to a decline in oxygen consumption. Other investigators have similarly pointed out the high incidence of cerebrovascular disease and the widened cerebral arteriovenous oxygen differences in the dementias of old age.[35, 40, 58] An alternative viewpoint was presented by Lassen and his colleagues[43] who argued that the reduced oxygen uptake could be explained by cortical atrophy and an endogenous decline in neuronal metabolism. The decreased blood flow would thus represent an intrinsic adjustment of the circulation to the lesser metabolic demands of the tissue. With either hypothesis, dementia rather than age is the critical variable associated with the decreased blood flow. The available evidence cannot help us decide between these alternatives. Both types of pathological processes, cerebral ischemia due to arteriosclerosis and parenchymatous neuronal degeneration, may contribute to the altered metabolic parameters in dementia.

An alternative approach is to suggest that certain neural structures and functions possess a low margin of safety. Under these circumstances, a variety of biochemical alterations may be present, but the important variable would be the overwhelming impairment of one particular facet of neural function. For example, studies of the amino-acidurias suggest that myelin alterations may explain altered mental function.[46] Regardless of which specific biochemical dysfunction brought about the condition, changes in function of the myelin sheath would be considered the final common pathway inducing the behavioral effects. Unfortunately, the evidence implicating myelin or any other structure as being particularly responsible for the dysfunction is far from convincing.

Another example of this approach might be to differentiate among various types of neurons and to suggest that one selected group might be particularly susceptible to a range of biochemical defects, such as hippocampal neurons are to anoxia. Any biochemical process that affects these critical neurons would thereby alter the communal response. Two different hypotheses could be entertained: (1) The severity of dementia is directly related to the gross amount of impaired cerebral tissue and the total quantitative loss of neurons, or (2) the dementia complex reflects neuronal loss in selected areas of the brain. Presumably both hypotheses have merit. The symptom complex of dementia with general loss of highest integrative function is most compatible with diffuse dysfunction. However, circumscribed focal involvement might give rise to components of the dementia complex such as bilateral impairment of limbic lobe function giving rise to memory disturbances.

A vital process such as neuronal-glial or neuronal-neuronal (synaptic) interaction rather than the total cell population might also have a low threshold for biochemical perturbations. In fact since the synapse is often a key and rate-limiting step in intercellular communication within the nervous system, alterations in the pattern of synaptic organization and the efficiency of synaptic function might well be reflected behaviorally as dementia.

The data are not available to choose correctly among these several alternatives. It seems likely that in many of the dementias both rate-limiting biochemical reactions and rate-limiting neuronal functions might contribute to the behavioral aberrations. Although neurons from different regions of the brain have different enzymatic constituents and are differentially susceptible to a range of metabolic deficiencies, present data suggest that dementia is best correlated with a total reduction in the number of functioning neurons, regardless of the specific biochemical defect.

RESEARCH APPROACHES TO DEMENTIA

Advances in the understanding of brain dysfunction in dementia have been derived from several sources: (1) Direct biochemical and morphological examination of the brain in a particular type of dementia, made possible by the increasing sophistication of electron microscopic techniques, the availability of suitable brain biopsy specimens, and the advances in understanding protein, nucleic acid, and lipid metabolism. (2) Investigation of the biochemistry of memory, employing inhibitors of protein and nucleic acid synthesis. (3) Empirical trials of a wide spectrum of drugs and natural products as adjuncts in the therapy of dementia. Despite these advances, the number of biochemical investigations of diseases presenting primarily with dementia is limited. Therapy is not yet based either upon a sound theoretical framework or upon well-documented biochemical defects.

Correlation of Pathological and Biochemical Changes

Senile Plaques

In the previous chapter three pathological changes were noted to be markedly increased in patients with presenile and senile dementia. These are senile plaques, neurofibrillary tangles, and granulovacuolar degeneration. By ultrastructural studies senile plaques were noted to consist of an extracellular core of fibrils resembling amyloid, surrounded by cytoplasmic processes containing fibrils, multilamellar bodies, and degenerating mitochondria.[63] In the region of senile plaques, changes in axons and presynaptic and postsynpaptic processes have been noted,[32, 44] and enzyme histochemistry demonstrated increased oxidative function, presumably representing an early metabolic reaction to neuronal injury, especially in the neuropil.[24, 25] The deposits were characterized as amyloid because they exhibited a carbohydrate-containing protein with dichromic birefringence when stained with Congo red. The filamentous material of senile plaques is extracellular and appears to possess the morphological appearance of amyloid noted in other conditions.[39, 64] The identification of amyloid in senile plaques has, however, shed little light on the etiology of primary dementias since (1) senile plaques are present in brains of old patients who exhibited no dementia (although such plaques are quantitatively less in such patients than in patients with Alzheimer's disease or senile dementia) ,[65] and (2) the central nervous system is very rarely involved in generalized amyloidosis.

Neurofibrillary Changes

The etiology of the neurofibrillary alterations and hippocampal pyramidal cell granulovacuolar bodies is unknown. They occur under a variety of conditions ranging from senile and presenile dementia to chronic encephalitis and mongolism, as well as being present in older individuals who never exhibited dementia (although such changes were noted in quantitatively smaller concentrations in such patients) .[65] The neurofibrillary tangles are argyrophilic and by electron microscopy they prove to be closely aggregated coarse neurofilaments in a parallel array.[63] They have been produced by intracerebral aluminum injections[19, 41] and by colchicine.[66] By cytochemistry there is a marked increase in mass with no changes in RNA content or base composition.[19] Questions regarding the specificity of neurofibrillary tangles for a given metabolic error, or neuronal malfunction, or even its specificity for dementia have not been definitively answered.

Biochemistry of Alzheimer's and Jakob-Creutzfeldt Disease

The most detailed biochemical investigations have been reported in Alzheimer's disease and Jakob-Creutzfeldt disease. In biopsies of three cases of Alzheimer's disease, Suzuki, Katzman, and Korey[59] noted a decrease in total protein and an increase in total lipid in gray matter, producing a change in the protein-to-lipid ratio when compared to controls. One possible explanation of these data might be a specific reduction in brain protein-synthesizing capacity. However, when a microsomal system was prepared from Alzheimer brain tissue and compared to controls, no significant differences in this capacity were observed.[60] The rate of lysine-^{14}C incorporation was equivalent in both, although protein synthesis with brain tissue from older patients was significantly less than with tissue from younger patients. Such studies still do not exclude the possibility that neuronal protein synthesis might be significantly impaired. Microsomes isolated from brain are derived from both glial and neuronal sources and have been demonstrated to synthesize proteins of glial origin in vitro.[53] The contribution of glial synthetic capacity might be increased to provide the enhanced neurofibrillary content, and these changes might offset a diminished neuronal synthesis. Techniques presently available to separate neurons from glia might answer the question more definitively.[50] In aluminum-induced experimental neurofibrillary degeneration, both the uptake of amino acid into neurofibrillary tangles and the RNA content are normal and

137

coincide with the findings in Alzheimer's disease.[19] In the absence of any specific evidence implicating either protein-synthesizing capacity or enhanced proteolytic activity in Alzheimer's disease, the decrease in total protein might be simply attributed to neuronal cell loss.[49] The techniques employed to date have not specified the biochemical defect in neurons in either experimentally induced or spontaneous neurofibrillary degeneration. Future detailed investigation in this area is essential. Perhaps analysis of changes at earlier periods might yield data relevant to the initial metabolic defect rather than to the complicated gliotic and reparative processes.

The biochemical analysis of the brain of a patient dying with Jakob-Creutzfeldt disease was the first to demonstrate glycolipid changes associated with dementia.[42] In this case formalin-fixed material was employed and was compared to control tissue similarly treated. The striking feature was a decrease in gray-matter gangliosides. However, since this material had been formalin fixed, the significance of this observation is unclear. Hexosamines were similarly reduced. In Alzheimer's disease total gangliosides have been noted to be reduced with chromatographic pattern of the various ganglioside species being identical in patients with dementia and controls.[59] Cherayil[12] and Cherayil and Cyrus[13] similarly noted a diminution in gangliosides with a normal distribution of subtypes.

Disagreement has been noted with respect to the cerebroside content in tissue of patients with Alzheimer's dementia. Suzuki[59] noted a marked increase in cerebrosides compared to controls, whereas Pope, Hess, and Lewin[49] and Rouser, aided by Galli and Kritchevsky[51, 52] in separate studies, observed a significant decrease. Rouser[52] also noted a change in the fatty acid composition of sphingomyelin and lecithin. The reason for the discrepancy in cerebrosides is not clear, although it may relate to differential sampling of gliotic areas and neurofibrillary tangles by different investigators. In brief, with the cases subjected to lipid analysis by various workers to date, there is no evidence of a specific biochemical defect that could not be explained merely on the basis of cell destruction or loss.

The presence of amyloid has been inferred from electron microscopic studies of senile plaques of tissue from patients with Alzheimer's disease.[32, 44, 51] In biopsies of three patients with Alzheimer's disease there was a twofold increase in acid mucopolysaccharides compared to control.[59] The chromatographic distribution of different acid mucopolysaccharide constituents was normal. Hyaluronic acid was the main mucopolysaccharide component as it is in the normal brain. There was no evidence of an abnormal mucopolysaccharide.

In brain biopsy specimens of patients with Alzheimer's disease, oxygen uptake, respiratory rate, lactic acid production, and glucose-^{14}C conversion to lipids and amino acid constituents were comparable to control brain tissue.[59]

In Huntington's chorea, decreased lipids and protein were found to be directly related to the cell loss of the caudate nucleus. Phospholipids were relatively decreased, but sphingomyelin was relatively increased. An increase in glutamic acid was the only change in amino acids.[8]

Potential Role of the Synapse in Dementia

Sampling the biochemical constituents of the entire biopsy specimen necessarily excludes specific analysis of neuronal, glial, or synaptic biochemistry. Therefore, it is possible that particular components of the nervous system, such as synaptic junctions, may be the primary but not yet detected site of the defect in dementia. It has been generally assumed that the synapse plays a secondary role and degenerates in a nonspecific manner following lesions of the perikaryon. Gonatas and Goldensohn,[32] however, have provided convincing evidence that synaptic pathological changes may be significant. Alterations in axonal and synaptic fine structure were demonstrated as the sole pathological finding in a patient with seizures, mental retardation, and cortical blindness, and a probable diagnosis of axonal dystrophy. Similar alterations consisting of enlargement of the presynaptic terminal, reduction of the number of synaptic vesicles, and accumulation of fibrillar and vesicular material were observed in biopsies of patients with Alzheimer's disease.[32] Multilamellar bodies were described in nerve endings in these biopsies. Such abnormalities in synaptic terminals might well cause disturbances in either transmitter output or the response of postsynaptic membranes, which might affect intercellular communication. Although these studies are not conclusive, they suggest the hypothesis that synaptic function represents a rate-limiting process in neuronal interaction and that impairment in any facet of such function may have widespread effects upon interneuronal interaction. Clearly any pathological process that prevented interneuronal communication would resemble a process that diffusely destroyed neurons.

Biochemistry of Memory

In no way do the previous studies exclude a specific biochemical effect giving rise to neuronal deterioration and diffuse dysfunction. Alterations may be present in membrane structure and function, specific enzymatic constituents of protein or carbohydrate metabolism, or critical cellular elements such as messenger RNA, which represent only a small percentage of the total species. Such biochemical disturbances would not have been detected by the analyses employed. The question must therefore be raised whether other studies of brain function implicate macromolecules in any significant way.

Recent advances in the biochemistry of memory and in the evaluation of nucleic acids and protein in such processes[30] appear relevant to an understanding of dementia, where memory loss is such a prominent feature. Recent progress in molecular biology has offered the theoretical basis for the coding of experience in macromolecules. With the important rate-limiting function demonstrated to exist for messenger RNA in bacterial systems, an analogy was sought with the memory engram.

139

Transfer of "Memory" with Macromolecules

Several hypotheses were proposed to explain how protein or nucleic acid macromolecules, or both, might be involved in memory storage. The code may be recorded either in the primary structure or in the composition of a set of macromolecules. Thus, correlation could be made between the presence of the macromolecules and the prior experience of the organism. A further implication of this theory would be that such molecules could be directly injected into the brain of a naive animal to create a specific bit of information. Unfortunately, no convincing evidence exists for the presence of a specific molecule that might appear with a given experience, last for the extent of that experience, disappear when recall or retrieval of that experience is no longer demonstrable, and reappear with the reappearance of the specific behavioral set. Although considerable speculation centers upon such a class of specific memory molecules, no direct reproducible evidence documents their existence, and we must maintain a healthy skepticism about this approach. The lack of reproducibility of transfer of information with RNA is not really surprising since intraperitoneally or orally administered RNA has never been shown to become incorporated into brain cells.[45] It is unlikely that such a large molecule could penetrate either the blood-brain barrier or brain cells without being broken down. These experiments do not exclude a role for RNA; they merely indicate that RNA may be only one component of the cellular response to stimuli, and that interanimal, interorgan, or even intercellular transfer of macromolecule RNA may not be a significant method for information transfer in the brain.

Network Approaches to "Memory"

Another possibility is that the experience is coded and recorded as the altered responsiveness of neural networks. The role of any macromolecular alterations associated with a change in experience and adaptation of the organism would be to enhance individual neuronal participation in a particular pathway. The new state could be merely an enhancement of the efficiency of interneuronal communication leading to more facile interneuronal transmission. The individual cell does not know whether it has participated in a learning experience or not. The individual neurons would merely have a greater or smaller likelihood of discharge. Only the final output of the neuronal network would convey the information of registration, storage, or retrieval. In such a scheme similar macromolecules could be used in many different cells for the purpose of enhancing information passage and transfer. Several ways by which cells could increase the efficiency of interneuronal communication would be to: (1) enhance the availability of neurotransmitter, (2) change the likelihood of transmitter release associated with presynaptic terminal depolarization, (3) narrow the intersynaptic cleft through which the transmitter must diffuse, or (4) alter the nature of the receptor site or the postsynaptic membrane responsiveness.

Alterations in RNA and Protein Associated with "Memory"

To many investigators a likely candidate to bring about such facilitation is the presence of a new protein or increased amounts of an existing protein constituent. Such proteins then would have unique effects altering the biochemistry of the synapse to give rise to the altered interneuronal communication. The proteins would be specified by an RNA synthesized in response to gene activation brought on by the learning experience. Evidence implicating RNA in such a process is of two types: (1) use of antimetabolites, which interfere with RNA synthesis and thereby either block the storage process or information retrieval, and (2) demonstration that a new species of RNA is associated with the acquisition of new information.

Antibiotics and Antimetabolites in the Study of Memory

Actinomycin D is a drug that blocks the transcription of DNA to form RNA macromolecules. The compound appears to have little effect on the stretch receptor of the crayfish or subsequent membrane potentials.[18] Furthermore, it has only a limited effect in blocking memory storage in mice[5, 14] although it does interfere significantly with such processes in the goldfish.[4] In the goldfish, following actinomycin D inhibition of RNA synthesis up to 70 per cent, profound memory deficits were demonstrated under conditions that did not prevent normal performance of the learned task. 8-Azaguanine, a purine antimetabolite, was thought to affect learning and not performance on a maze water problem.[56] The specific effects of RNA metabolism on performance are not clear, however, and psychological parameters suggested depression of motor activity as an explanation for the observed behavioral changes.[11]

Increased RNA Associated with Learning and Memory

Observations of whether learning and memory are associated with increased RNA represent an alternative way to study the importance of RNA. The difficulty in such experiments is the usual lack of adequate controls for the specific stresses that an animal undergoes while training. Adair, Wilson, Zemp, and Glassman[2] and Adair, Wilson, and Glassman[1] carefully attempted to control for such nonspecific factors. They demonstrated that mice trained for 15 minutes to avoid a shock by jumping to a shelf incorporate 50 per cent more radioactive uridine into brain RNA and polysomes than untrained mice yoked to the trained ones. Such enhanced incorporation was not seen in liver or kidney RNA and appeared to be most marked in subcortical areas, especially the diencephalon, whereas decreased incorporation into RNA was demonstrated in the cortex.

The experiments of Hyden and his co-workers focus on changes in nuclear RNA associated with the training process.[36, 38] His experiments demonstrate that increased stimulation is associated with elevation of the RNA levels, and the particular type of training experience appears to have differential effects on the base ratios observed. These experiments have been criticized, both with respect to the psychological parameters employed and the interpretation of the base ratio shifts.

Hyden and Egyhazi[36] reported that during passive stimulation the RNA content of the neuron increased but that of the glial cell fell, whereas in learning both neuronal and glial RNA increased. Hyden and Lange[37] suggested that early in learning a DNA-like RNA is made in responding nerve cells and that after the animal has learned, a ribosomal-like RNA is produced. Although the data are compatible with such an interpretation, further confirmation is necessary since other interpretations could equally well be drawn from the reported experiments.

Inhibitors of Protein Synthesis and Information Transfer

The nature of the consolidation process leading to long-term memory has also been studied by the use of drugs that inhibit protein synthesis. But as with RNA, the role of protein synthesis is uncertain. In investigations with puromycin, Flexner, Flexner and Stellar[20] demonstrated that injections of quantities that inhibit over 90 per cent of protein synthesis were associated with significant impairment in information retrieval or storage. Injections of puromycin into the temporal-hippocampal region produced an interference with memory lasting several days. However, combined injections into the temporal, hippocampal, caudal, frontal, and periventricular regions were necessary 11 to 43 days after training to impair storage. Furthermore, acetoxycycloheximide, another inhibitor of protein synthesis, prevented the memory impairment when given simultaneously with puromycin.[21] Flexner, Flexner, and Roberts[23] also postulated that proteins involved in the maintenance and expression of memory act as inducers of the synthesis of their own messenger RNA and that puromycin acts by accelerating the destruction of this messenger RNA so that both the proteins and memory are lost.

Several significant objections have been raised to these interpretations: (1) Injections of saline alone reverse the memory deficit, thereby implicating some product of puromycin independent of its effect on protein synthesis or messenger RNA.[22] (2) Puromycin alters hippocampal electrical activity, and the electrical changes and behavioral effects can be reversed by anticonvulsants.[15] (3) Puromycin causes marked alterations in the morphology of neuronal mitochondria and could potentially alter neuronal energy metabolism.[26] All of the results may be explained by the presence of a puromycyl peptide, which may interfere with membrane function and thereby produce the observed effects.

In studies by Barondes and Cohen[7] and Agranoff, Davis, and Brink[3] acetoxycycloheximide has been demonstrated to impair long-term memory without depressing brain activity, since mice and goldfish readily relearn the task that they could not recall and show no performance deficit. The amount of training is critical to achieve an effect from acetoxycycloheximide.[7] If criterion is 9 out of 10, no effect can be demonstrated, whereas if criterion is 3 out of 4, a significant memory deficit can be demonstrated starting at 6 hours after train-ing and lasting for at least 7 days. These data suggest the potential importance of inhibition of protein synthesis in the study of memory. Unfortunately, in mice, puromycin can no longer be used as a control for acetoxycycloheximide because of its independent effects upon mitochondrial function. No other pro-tein synthesis inhibitor has been employed to strengthen the argument that protein synthesis inhibition per se is the critical variable and not some yet-to-be discovered side effect of acetoxycycloheximide.

It is well established that stimulation and nerve activity can cause changes in RNA and proteins of the nerve cell. The evidence, however, that RNA and proteins are directly involved in storage and memory is at present cir-cumstantial. Chemical changes can be demonstrated during learning, but their primary associations with stress, activity, or stimulation rather than memory storage must be questioned. Perhaps the most critical factor is that no data are available to indicate the role of the responding chemical in neural function or to indicate any causal relationship between the behavioral and the chemical change. The possibility exists that such chemical changes may be unrelated responses to separate components of the same experience.

Drugs and Natural Products in Dementia

The evidence implicating neural proteins in learning and memory is more convincing than that implicating nucleic acids, though use of the latter has represented a major effort to enhance performance in man. The theoretical premise employed is that if diminutions in RNA are associated with im-paired performance, increases in neural RNA might be associated with im-proved performance. Some of the initial attempts in this area were performed with yeast RNA or nucleotides. In the studies of Cameron, Solym, and Beach,[10] patients with diagnoses of arteriosclerotic, senile, presenile dementia and Korsakoff's psychosis were given approximately 700 gm. of yeast RNA over a 12-week period and evaluated by a variety of different tests. Unfor-tunately, no satisfactory controls were provided, and the range of improve-ment reported may have been due to a variety of causes unrelated to the par-ticular substance being administered. Indeed, Nodine and associates[47], were unsuccessful in several attempts at reproducing Cameron's results using a double-blind technique. Similar experiments have been reported in rats by Cook and co-workers,[16] who demonstrated that the administration of yeast RNA nucleotides enhanced acquisition and delayed extinction of a condi-tioned avoidance response. Two potential explanations of positive results might be offered: (1) RNA or nucleotides may possess intrinsic information, and (2) the brain does not have adequate pools of nucleotide precursors and cannot synthesize the molecules de novo; thus, the RNA or nucleotides would

143

represent a nutritional supplement. Luttges and his group[45] have demonstrated convincingly that intraperitoneal RNA does not enter the brain in detectable amounts, and it appears unlikely that the administered nucleotides carry any specific information. On the other hand, Geiger and Yamasaki[27] demonstrated the dependence of the isolated perfused cat's brain upon circulating uridine and cytidine. Our data also suggest that the brain may not synthesize nucleotides de novo and therefore may depend upon endogenous and exogenous nucleotides as precursors for RNA synthesis and as cofactors for mucopolysaccharide, glycoprotein, and lipid synthesis.[6]

Long-term administration of tricyanoaminopropane (TCAP) has been demonstrated to facilitate maze learning in rats.[54] In one report, bright rats were unaffected by TCAP, but dull rats showed greatly improved learning.[17] In both situations it was difficult to ascertain whether positive effects were due to increased RNA synthesis or stimulant effects of the drug. When geriatric patients were given the drug in a control study, it failed to enhance favorable practice effects and showed some tendency to depress them.[62] When mice were injected with TCAP, there appeared to be a definite performance facilitation which was correlated with enhanced RNA content.[55] However, as previously noted, stimulation itself may give rise to such increases in RNA; and there is no evidence for a specific alteration in information acquisition, storage, or retrieval.

Magnesium pemoline, which is a combination of 2-imino-5-phenyl-4-oxazolidinone and magnesium hydroxide, produced considerable excitement among physicians and investigators when it was initially suggested to have a specific effect on memory and learning.[9] Glasky and Simon[29] reported the drug increased RNA polymerase activity of rat brain in vivo and in vitro, but these studies have not been confirmed. In general, the behavioral effects of the drug are not clear.[31] A facilitation of learning has either not been confirmed or has been ascribed to stimulant effects or to increased sensitivity to shock, both of which may produce an apparent facilitation of learning.[34] In humans, Cameron[9] reported a statistically significant increase in intelligence in senile patients given 25 to 40 mg. of magnesium pemoline daily for at least 1 month, but psychometric data are lacking and the placebo effects were not controlled. No effects were noted when single doses up to 37 mg. of magnesium pemoline were administered to college students. The data of Talland[61] would suggest that the compound is a general stimulant, and either this or its anti-fatigue action is primarily responsible for the altered performance.

It is clear that therapies of dementia based on an enhancement of nucleic acid synthesis and levels have at best provided stimulant effects on performance. Nevertheless, these results are important because they suggest that despite tissue degeneration, remaining viable neurons may possibly be made to perform in a more efficient manner. It is not clear whether the use of such stimulants may make excessive cellular energy demands and thereby compromise neuronal longevity.

CONCLUSIONS

The main result of the experiments on memory has been to emphasize how little we know about the biochemistry of mental function. Analyses of changes in RNA turnover, protein synthesis, and lipid constituents tell us little about the subcellular changes that take place. The critical element is the tight coupling of membrane function with intracellular metabolism and the interaction of many exquisitely regulated neurons. The data suggest that neuronal loss best correlates with the presence of dementia and that no unique biochemical event or deficiency can explain dementia.

In general, the biochemical data provided by animal investigations of learning and memory are an inadequate base at the present time to devise rational therapies for the treatment of patients with dementia. The concept of alterations in protein and nucleic acid synthesis holds some promise in developing hypotheses to understand both short- and long-term memory and neuronal alterations in the dementias. Unfortunately, to date such hypotheses have not led to a sound theoretical framework to treat the memory disorders of dementia.

Lacking any sound chemical theory for dementia, it might be equally rewarding to concentrate on a particular process that may be positively or negatively affected by the increases or decreases in a particular macromolecular constituent. Synaptic function, being the key or rate-limiting event in brain information processing, may well be such a process. Numerous theories of the biochemistry of memory postulate that a long-lasting change in macromolecular constituents is primarily earmarked for altering synaptic function. If one could demonstrate that pathology exists in the synapse in association with dementia, it would give a clue that alterations in synaptic function are the sine qua non of dementia. Any pathological process that prevented interneuronal communication would resemble a process that diffusely destroyed neurons. Even the precision of the electron microscope may not be able to define the range of alterations in synaptic function that may give rise to the dementias. Changes in transmitter synthesis and release, membrane structure, coupling between receptor-transmitter interactions and membrane depolarization are beyond the resolution of the electron microscope; yet any of these are conceivable early changes of both primary and secondary dementias.

The biochemical approaches to such problems are in their infancy, but further investigations in these areas should prove extremely fruitful.

REFERENCES

1. ADAIR, L. B., WILSON, J. E., AND GLASSMAN, E.: *Brain function and macromolecules. IV. Uridine incorporation into polysomes of mouse brain during different behavioral experiences.* Proc. Nat. Acad. Sci. 61:917, 1968.

2. ADAIR, L. B., WILSON, J. E., ZEMP, J. W., AND GLASSMAN, E.: *Brain function and macromolecules. III. Uridine incorporation into polysomes of mouse brain during short-term avoidance conditioning.* Proc. Nat. Acad. Sci. 61:606, 1968.

3. AGRANOFF, B. W., DAVIS, R. E., AND BRINK, J. J.: *Chemical studies on memory fixation in goldfish.* Brain Res. 1:303, 1966.

4. AGRANOFF, B. W., DAVIS, R. E., CASOLA, L., ET AL.: *Actinomycin-D blocks formation of memory of shock-avoidance in goldfish.* Science 158:1600, 1967.

5. APPEL, S. H.: *The effect of inhibition of RNA synthesis on neural information.* Nature 207:1163, 1965.

6. APPEL, S. H., AND SILBERBERG, D.: *Pyrimidine synthesis in tissue culture.* J. Neurochem. 15:1437, 1968.

7. BARONDES, S. H., AND COHEN, H. D.: *Delayed and sustained effect of acetoxycycloheximide on memory in mice.* Proc. Nat. Acad. Sci. 58:157, 1967.

8. BORRI, P. F., OP DEN VELDE, W. M., HOOGHWINKEL, G. J. M., AND BRUYN, G. W.: *Biochemical studies in Huntington's chorea. VI. Composition of striatal neutral lipids, phospholipids, glycolipids, fatty acids and amino acids.* Neurology 17:172, 1967.

9. CAMERON, D. E.: *Magnesium pemoline and human performance.* Science 157:958, 1967.

10. CAMERON, D. E., SOLYM, L., AND BEACH, L.: *Further studies upon the effects of the administration of ribonucleic acid in aged patients suffering from memory (retention) failure.* Neuropsychopharmacology 2:351, 1961.

11. CHAMBERLAIN, T. J., ROTHSCHILD, G. H., AND GERARD, R. W.: *Drugs affecting RNA and learning.* Proc. Nat. Acad. Sci. 49:918, 1961.

12. CHERAYIL, G. D.: *Fatty acid composition of brain glycolipids in Alzheimer's disease, senile dementia, and cerebrocortical atrophy.* J. Lipid Res. 9: 207, 1968.

13. CHERAYIL, G. D., AND CYRUS, A. E., JR.: *The quantitative estimation of glycolipids in Alzheimer's disease.* J. Neurochem. 13:579, 1966.

14. COHEN, H. D., AND BARONDES, S. H.: *Further studies of learning and memory after intracerebral actinomycin-D.* J. Neurochem. 13:207, 1966.

15. COHEN, H. D., ERVIN, F., AND BARONDES, S. H.: *Puromycin and cycloheximide: Different effects on hippocampal electrical activity.* Science 154: 1557, 1966.

16. COOK, L., DAVIDSON, A., DAVIS, D., GREEN, H., AND FELLOWS, E. J.: *Ribonucleic acid: Effect on conditioned behavior in rats.* Science 144:268, 1963.

17. DANIELS, D.: *The effect of TCAP in acquisition of discrimination learning in the rat.* Psychon. Sci. 7:5, 1967.

18. EDSTROM, J. E., AND GRAMPP, W.: *Nervous activity and metabolism of ribonucleic acids in the Crustacean stretch receptor neuron.* J. Neurochem. 12:735, 1965.

19. EMBREE, L. J., HAMBERGER, A., AND SJOSTRAND, J.: *Quantitative cytochemical studies and histochemistry in experimental neurofibrillary degeneration.* J. Neuropath. Exp. Neurol. 26:427, 1967.

20. FLEXNER, J. B., FLEXNER, L. B. AND STELLAR, E.: *Memory in mice as affected by intracerebral puromycin.* Science 141:57, 1963.

21. FLEXNER, L. B. AND FLEXNER, J. B.: *Effect of acetoxycycloheximide and of an acetoxycycloheximide-puromycin mixture on cerebral protein synthesis and "memory" in mice.* Proc. Nat. Acad. Sci. 55:369, 1966.

22. FLEXNER, L. B., AND FLEXNER, J. B.: *Intracerebral saline: Effect on memory of trained mice treated with puromycin.* Science 159:330, 1968.

23. FLEXNER, L. B., FLEXNER, J. B. AND ROBERTS, R. B.: *Stages of memory in mice treated with acetoxycycloheximide before or immediately after learning.* Proc. Nat. Acad. Sci. 56:730, 1966.

24. FRIEDE, R. L.: *Enzyme histochemical studies of senile plaques.* J. Neuropath. Exp. Neurol. 24:477, 1965.

25. FRIEDE, R. L., AND MAGEE, K. R.: *Alzheimer's disease. Presentation of a case with pathologic and enzymatic histochemical observations.* Neurology 12:213, 1962.

26. GAMBETTI, P. L., GONATAS, N. K., AND FLEXNER, L. B.: *The fine structure of puromycin-induced changes in mouse entorhinal cortex.* J. Cell Biol. 35:379, 1968.

27. GEIGER, A., AND YAMASAKI, S.: *Cytidine and uridine requirements of the brain.* J. Neurochem. 1:93, 1956.

28. GIBBS, C. J., JR., GAJDUSEK, D. C., ASHER, D. M., ALPERS, M. P., BECK, E., DANIEL, P. M., AND MATTHEWS, W. M.: *Creutzfeldt-Jakob disease (spongiform encephalopathy): Transmission to the chimpanzee.* Science 161: 388, 1968.

29. GLASKY, A. J., AND SIMON, L. N.: *Magnesium pemoline: Enhancement of brain RNA polymerases.* Science 151:702, 1966.

30. GLASSMAN, E.: *The biochemistry of learning: An evaluation of the role of RNA and protein.* Ann. Rev. Biochem. 38:605, 1969.

31. GOLDBERG, M. E., AND CIOFALO, V. B.: *Failure of magnesium pemoline to enhance acquisition of the avoidance response in mice.* Life Sci. 6:733, 1967.

32. GONATAS, N. K., ANDERSON, W., AND EVANGELISTA, I.: *The contribution of altered synapses in the senile plaque: An electron microscopic study in Alzheimer's dementia.* J. Neuropath. Exp. Neurol. 26:25, 1967.

33. GONATAS, N. K., AND GOLDENSOHN, E. S.: *Unusual neocortical presynaptic terminals in a patient with convulsions, mental retardation, and cortical blindness: An electron microscopic study.* J. Neuropath. Exp. Neurol. 24:539, 1965.

34. GUROWITZ, E. M., LUBAR, J. R., AIN, B. R., AND GROSS, D. A.: *Disruption of passive avoidance learning by magnesium pemoline.* Psychon. Sci. 8:19, 1967.

35. HASSLER, O.: *Vascular changes in senile brains.* Acta Neuropath. (Berl.) 5:40, 1965.

36. HYDEN, H., AND EGYHAZI, E.: *Glial RNA changes during a learning experiment in rats.* Proc. Nat. Acad. Sci. 49:618, 1963.

37. HYDEN, H., AND LANGE, P. W.: *A differentiation in RNA response in neurons early and late during learning.* Proc. Nat. Acad. Sci. 53:946, 1965.

38. HYDEN, H., AND LANGE, P. W.: *Protein synthesis in the hippocampal pyramidal cells of rats during a behavioral test.* Science 159:1370, 1968.

39. KATZMAN, R., AND SUZUKI, K.: *A search for a chemical correlate of amyloid in senile plaques of Alzheimer's disease.* Trans. Amer. Neurol. Assn. 89:17, 1964.

40. KETY, S. S.: *Human cerebral blood flow and oxygen consumption as related to aging.* Res. Publ. Assn. Nerv. Ment. Dis. 35:31, 1956.

41. KLATZO, I., WISNIEWSKI, H., AND STREICHER, E.: *Experimental production of neurofibrillary degeneration. I. Light microscopic observation.* J. Neuropath. Exp. Neurol. 24:187, 1965.

42. KOREY, S. R., KATZMAN, R., AND ORLOFF, J.: *A case of Jakob-Creutzfeldt disease.* J. Neuropath. Exp. Neurol. 20:95, 1961.

43. LASSEN, N. A., FEINBERG, I., AND LANE, M. H.: *Bilateral studies of cerebral oxygen uptake in young and aged normal subjects and in patients with organic dementia.* J. Clin. Invest. 39:491, 1960.

44. LUSE, S. A., AND SMITH, K. R.: *The ultrastructure of senile plaques.* Amer. J. Path. 44:553, 1964.

45. LUTTGES, M., JOHNSON, T., BUCK, C. HOLLAND, J., AND McGAUGH, J.: *An examination of "transfer of learning" by nucleic acid.* Science 151: 834, 1966.

46. MENKES, J. H.: *The pathogenesis of mental retardation in phenylketonuria and other inborn errors of amino acid metabolism.* Pediatrics 39: 397, 1967.

47. NODINE, J. H., SHULKIN, M. W., SLAP, J. W., LEVINE, M., AND FREIBERG, K.: *A double-blind study of the effect of ribonucleic acid in senile brain disease.* Amer. J. Psychiat. 123:1257, 1966.

48. OBRIST, W. D., CHIVIAN, E., CRONQUIST, S., AND INGVAR, D. H.: *Regional cerebral blood flow in senile and presenile dementia.* Neurology 20:315, 1970.

49. POPE, A., HESS, H., AND LEWIN, E.: *Microchemical pathology of the cerebral cortex in presenile dementias.* Trans. Amer. Neurol. Assn. 89:15, 1964.

50. ROSE, S. P. R.: *Preparation of enriched fractions from cerebral cortex containing isolated metabolically active neuronal cells.* Nature 206:621, 1965.

51. ROUSER, G.: *Speculations on the nature of the metabolic defects in Tay-Sachs, Nieman-Pick, Gaucher's and Alzheimer's disease, and metachromatic leukodystrophy.* J. Amer. Oil Chem. Soc. 42:412, 1965.

52. ROUSER, G., GALLI, C., AND KRITCHEVSKY, G.: *Lipid class composition of normal human brain and variations in metachromatic leukodystrophy, Tay-Sachs, Nieman-Pick, chronic Gaucher's and Alzheimer's disease.* J. Amer. Oil Chem. Soc. 42:404, 1965.

53. RUBIN, A. L., AND STENZEL, K. H.: *In vitro synthesis of brain protein.* Proc. Nat. Acad. Sci. 53:963, 1965.

54. SCHMIDT, M. J., AND DAVENPORT, J. W.: *TCAP: Facilitation of learning in hypothryoid rats.* Psychon. Sci. 7:185, 1967.

55. SEITE, R., CHAMBOST, G., AND DURAND, S.: *Influence du tricyanoamino-propane sur l'activite elaborairice des neurones ganglionnaires vegetatifs chez le chat.* Compt. Rend. Soc. Biol. 158:577, 1964.

56. SINGMAN, W., AND SPORN, M. B.: *The incorporation of 8-azaguanine into rat brain RNA and its effect on maze-learning by the rat: An inquiry into the biochemical basis of memory.* J. Psychiat. Res. 1:1, 1961.

57. SKINHOJ, E.: *Regulation of cerebral blood flow as a single function of the interstitial pH in the brain.* Acta Neurol. Scand. 42:604, 1966.

58. SOKOLOFF, L.: *Cerebral circulatory and metabolic changes associated with aging.* Res. Publ. Assn. Nerv. Ment. Dis. 41:237, 1966.

59. SUZUKI, K., KATZMAN, R., AND KOREY, S. R.: *Chemical studies on Alz-heimer's disease.* J. Neuropath. Exp. Neurol. 24:211, 1965.

60. SUZUKI, K., KOREY, S. R., AND TERRY, R. D.: *Studies on protein synthesis in brain microsomal system.* J. Neurochem. 11:403, 1964.

61. TALLAND, G. A.: *Improvement of sustained attention with cylert.* Psychon. Sci. 6:493, 1966.

62. TALLAND, G. A., MENDELSON, J. H., KOZ, G., AND AARON, R.: *Experimental studies of the effects of tricyanoaminopropane on the memory and learning capacities of geriatric patients.* J. Psychiat. Res. 3:171, 1965.

63. TERRY, R. D.: *The fine structure of neurofibrillary tangles in Alzheimer's disease.* J. Neuropath. Exp. Neurol. 22:629, 1963.

64. TERRY, R. D., GONATAS, N. K., AND WEISS, M.: *Ultrastructural studies in Alzheimer's presenile dementia.* Amer. J. Pathol. 44:269, 1964.

65. TOMLINSON, B. E., BLESSED, G., AND ROTH, M.: *Observations on the brain of non-demented old people.* J. Neurol. Sci. 7:331, 1968.

66. WISNIEWSKI, H., AND TERRY, R. D.: *Further studies on experimental neurofibrillary tangles.* J. Neuropath. Exp. Neurol. 27:149, 1968.

Chapter 9

Dementia in Old Age

H. Shan Wang, M.B., and
Ewald W. Busse, M.D.

Dementia is one of the most common clinical syndromes among aged persons. About 63 per cent of the elderly persons who are currently institutionalized in all public and private psychiatric hospitals and nursing homes in the United States have dementia.[29] Thus, out of every 100,000 elderly persons of age 65 years or over in the population, 2300 may have dementia of such severity that institutional care is necessary.

Dementia, though probably of less severity, is also quite common among elderly persons in the community. In fact the prominent effect of age on intellectual function is so well recognized that most objective measures for the assessment of intellectual function are constructed with a correction factor for age. Younger persons are given an age debit; older ones, an age credit. Take, for example, the Wechsler Adult Intelligence Scale (WAIS) —the most widely used psychological measure for intellectual function. A 25-year-old person has to obtain a verbal score of 60 or a performance of 50 in order to be classified as having an I.Q. of 100, the mean value of U.S. population. In contrast, the corresponding values are, respectively, 56 and 37 for a person 60 years old, 44 and 25 for a person over 74 years old. In other words, an average old person is expected to have a verbal ability 7 to 27 per cent below and a performance ability 26 to 50 per cent below that of an average adult. Wechsler[32] summarized: "Every human capacity after initial growth attains a maximum and then begins to decline. This decline is at first very slow but after a while increases perceptibly. The age at which the maximum is attained varies from ability to ability but seldom occurs beyond 30 and in most cases somewhere in the mid-20's. Once the decline begins, it progresses uninterruptedly. Between the ages of 30 and 60 it is more or less linear."

The intellectual decline of old age usually follows a certain pattern. Verbal abilities and stored information show relatively little, if any, deficit; while psychomotor skills, especially those involving speed and perceptual-integrative abilities, decline much more appreciably.[4] The correlation between age and performance abilities is therefore greater than that between age and verbal abilities. Consequently, with advancing age, there is also an increasing discrepancy between verbal and performance abilities which has often been used as an indicator of dementia.

THE VALIDITY OF AGE TREND OF INTELLECTUAL DETERIORATION

There are some questions about the validity and, particularly, the implication of these generalizations concerning the intellectual decline in old age. One common criticism is that these generalizations are derived mainly from cross-sectional studies that probably have exaggerated the pattern of decline in old age.[12] Cross-sectional studies reveal only age differences that could well be the result of a difference in education and sociocultural background between generations. Using a battery of neuropsychological tests that is independent of education, Halstead[13] has shown that 78 per cent of a group of high-level executives, averaging 50 years in age, could perform as well as a group of medical students of much younger ages. Longitudinal studies, on the other hand, can demonstrate more clearly the changes with age, but so far there have been only a few such reports on elderly persons.[2,12,14,21] According to these studies, the intellectual function of healthy elderly persons shows no significant decline over a period of 1 to 3 years. For a longer interval such as 5 to 8 years, the intellectual decline for a group of elderly persons becomes more obvious. Nevertheless, there are considerable individual variations within the group. Birren[2] reported that among 29 healthy elderly persons retested after 5 years, 5 or 17 per cent showed slight gain or no change in their WAIS performance. This is confirmed by another longitudinal study.[31] Among 32 community volunteers who had 12 or more years of education and whose good health was maintained for at least 3 to 4 years, 53 per cent showed either an increase or no change in their WAIS verbal scores. The corresponding figure for performance was 41 per cent. Although the absence of decline on repeated psychological assessment may be attributable in part to a practice or learning effect, these findings nevertheless indicate that intellectual deterioration does not occur in every old person and that it is not a gradual or linear process correlated with age. For most elderly persons, intellectual function may remain almost unchanged for some time during senescence and then decline more perceptibly, most likely in association with declining health or impending death.

THE ROLE OF THE BRAIN IN DEMENTIA

Why do some old persons become demented and others, though of comparable age, remain intellectually almost intact? If intellectual activities are the behavorial expression of brain activities, a close relationship should be expected to exist between the degree of dementia and the degree of brain impairment. Data so far available in this regard are contradictory, although a review of the literature[28] indicates that more often than not such a relationship can be demonstrated. Thus elderly persons with dementia generally manifest slowing of the electroencephalogram (EEG); they tend to show a greater reduction in their cerebral oxygen consumption and cerebral blood flow than the elderly whose mental abilities are preserved; and they have more senile plaque formation and more cerebral atrophy at postmortem examination.

EEG studies reveal considerable change with increasing age; even among elderly subjects in apparently good health, EEG abnormalities are common.[30] The characteristic abnormalities of the EEG's of senescent subjects are slowing of the dominant frequency and the appearance of focal defects, particularly over the left anterior temporal region. The slowing of the dominant rhythm is probably a reflection of depression of cerebral metabolism (see below). The significance of the focal defects is unclear, but they are frequent, beginning to appear even in middle age.

EEG's and WAIS scores were obtained on 27 elderly subjects living in the community with two examinations carried out 3.5 years apart.[31] Although there was considerable individual variation, no statistically significant change in verbal or performance scores was demonstrated between the two evaluations, nor was there a significant decrease in the frequency of the occipital alpha rhythm. When the data were evaluated for the individual subjects, however, there was a significant association between slower occipital EEG frequencies and lower verbal and performance scores on the WAIS. Slower frequencies on initial examination were also associated with a greater decline in both verbal and performance scores on the second examination. The frequency and prominence of EEG abnormalities in patients with known dementing illness is well established (see Chapter 5).

Both cerebral oxygen consumption and cerebral blood flow tend to decline in old age.[24] Early studies, though, compared groups of patients in which age was the only significant variable evaluated. In later studies, Dastur and associates[10] showed elderly subjects in good mental and physical health to have little if any decline in cerebral oxygen consumption and cerebral blood flow from that found in healthy younger subjects. On the other hand, cerebral oxygen consumption has been found reduced in the presence of organic dementia in both young and old subjects.[7] In a longitudinal study of healthy elderly subjects in which socioeconomic status and education were carefully controlled, those subjects who showed the greatest decline in their performance ability on the WAIS over an interval of 3 or more years tended to have low cerebral blood flow.[31]

The number of senile plaques found in the brain at postmortem examination generally increases with age.[1,25] Tomlinson, Blessed, and Roth[26] have demonstrated the presence of brain alterations usually seen in senile dementia (senile plaques, Alzheimer's neurofibrillary changes, granulovacuolar degeneration) in the brains of nondemented old people. The mere presence of these changes does not imply the presence of dementia; further studies,[3] however, in which the factor of age was controlled, have demonstrated "a very highly significant association between the average number of plaques in cerebral grey matter and measures of intellectual and personality functioning in old age. . . ." Other studies also confirm the relationship between the degree of brain atrophy (and pathological alterations) and the severity of intellectual and social disintegration.[9,33]

OUTCOME OF DEMENTIA

Elderly persons with severe dementia have many difficulties leading an independent life in the community; their management in an average family situation is likewise not easy. The result is the large number of elderly persons with dementia admitted for institutional care each year. It is estimated that about 36,000 elderly persons age 65 years or over, who had no previous psychiatric hospitalization, were admitted for the first time to a public or private mental hospital during the year of 1966.[29] Dementia accounted for about 78 per cent of all these first admissions during that year. As a rule, those patients admitted to a mental hospital who had clinical evidence of dementia or EEG evidence of brain impairment either had a high mortality or required long periods of institutionalization. For example, in a study of a group of elderly patients 2 years after admission, Trier[27] found that 33 per cent of those diagnosed as having dementia were still in the hospital and 57 per cent had died. Long-term hospitalization and death were much higher in this group than for a corresponding group having only psychogenic disorders. Only 9 per cent of patients with dementia were discharged from the hospital and could remain in the community at the end of the 2-year period.

In contrast to these generally gloomy predictions, the findings from a longitudinal project at the Duke Center for the Study of Aging and Human Development support the notion that at least some aged persons with dementia can remain in the community, leading a relatively active life. Between 1955 and 1959, 260 community volunteers above the age of 60 were recruited for long-term evaluation and study. Each subject who entered the study was evaluated initially by very thorough clinical and laboratory examinations administered by a multidisciplinary team. This thorough evaluation has since been repeated regularly at intervals of 3 or 4 years. Among these 260 community volunteers, about one third show either diffuse or focal disturbance in their EEG.[29] The cerebral blood flow of some subjects, as determined by the xenon-inhalation method, was less than one half of the value for normal young adults.[31] Some of the volunteers showed a 20 to 40 per cent decline in their test performance on the WAIS.[31] Nevertheless, over an interval of 12 years, though many of the subjects died, only one required hospitalization in a psychiatric institution. Quite a few, despite impaired brain function, impaired brain metabolism, and intellectual deterioration, were still capable of living an independent life in the community.

OTHER CONTRIBUTORY OR COMPLICATING FACTORS IN DEMENTIA

The relationship between dementia and brain status has not been consistently observed and even in those studies in which such a relationship has been demonstrated, discrepancies still occur in about one quarter of cases. In Corsellis'[9] study, 20 per cent of patients diagnosed as having senile psychosis showed no or little senile plaque formation on postmortem histopathological examination, while moderate to severe senile plaque formation was present in 9 per cent of patients having so-called functional psychosis. Discrepancies between senile plaque frequency and intellectual and social deterioration have also been observed by Blessed, Tomlinson, and Roth.[3] Willanger and co-workers[33] did not find significant evidence of dementia in 22 per cent of their subjects showing marked cerebral atrophy on pneumoencephalography. Although they encountered no patient with severe intellectual impairment without cerebral atrophy, the degree of atrophy was sometimes much less than would be anticipated from the result of psychological testing. Obrist and Henry[20] also noted that about one third of their patients diagnosed as having presenile or senile dementia had a cerebral blood flow within the normal range of healthy young adults. It is not uncommon for demented patients to have normal EEG's while psychologically well-preserved patients may have gross EEG abnormalities.[6,20]

The reliability and sensitivity of the methods employed in these studies unquestionably account for some of the discrepancies observed. It is well known that intellectual function and particularly its assessment, by clinical examination or by psychological test, are susceptible to the influence of many factors.[4] Few studies on dementia have paid attention to the sociocultural background of the subjects, although these sociocultural factors are known to bear on intellectual function as well as on certain brain variables such as the EEG.[30] Considerable evidence indicates that many somatic, psychological, and social factors participate in the development, manifestation, and outcome of dementia.

Somatic Factors

About three of every four persons 65 years old or over have at least one disabling chronic condition. Furthermore, each illness, once developed, usually lasts longer in elderly persons than in young adults.[8] Many diseases commonly associated with senescence affect the brain adversely. Elderly persons with cardiovascular disease, for example, have a high incidence of EEG abnormality[18] and many of them show a great decline in intellectual function.[11] Physical illness can directly impair brain tissue on which the intellectual activities depend. Willanger and his co-workers[33] noted that, with a given degree of cerebral atrophy, older persons showed greater intellectual impairment than younger ones. This finding suggests that the compensatory capacity of the remaining uninvolved brain tissue may be different in the two groups, a difference possibly attributable to a difference in physical health. Social inactivity or isolation, a common sequel to most chronic illnesses, frequently leads to psychological regression and depression, which contribute to and complicate the intellectual deterioration in old age.

Psychological Factors

Among the many psychological factors that are believed to bear on the intellectual deterioration of senescence, premorbid personality and depression are perhaps the two most important.

PREMORBID PERSONALITY.   In discussing his negative result on the relationship between clinical manifestations and pathological findings of the brain, Rothschild[23] considered the discrepancy between these two variables to be the result of a difference in mental compensatory mechanism. Kiev and his co-workers[16] found that patients who demonstrated a high order of adaptive versatility before their illness had less intellectual impairment in relation to loss of brain tissue than those who had for some time exhibited difficulties in overall adaptation with much anxiety. This is consistent with the observation that there seems to be a positive association between compulsive traits and dementia.[17] A compulsive person generally has a high expectation of himself and a strong need to control his relationship with others and with his environment. He generally reacts with excessive anxiety when his ability to control is threatened or jeopardized, as by a decline in his memory or other intellectual functions.

Anxiety of varying severity occurs in most elderly persons when they first become aware of their intellectual impairment. When under stress, these elderly persons may show the same type of psychic responses as do younger patients with brain damage.[15] Some may try to deny the defect; others avoid facing tasks or situations that provoke anxiety, or seek a substitute task or situation with which they believe they can cope; yet others become more rigid and compulsively orderly. The mechanisms preferred by each individual are frequently those most familiar to the individual and hence usually related closely to his premorbid personality.

When an aged person fails to relieve or alleviate the anxiety arising from interactions with his environment he tends to give up or avoid anxiety-provoking activities. Occasionally an aged person may become very aggressive in an attempt to control or manipulate his environment. This approach, however, frequently leads to his further alienation. As the elderly individual becomes more and more withdrawn or disengaged from society, the opportunity for his emotional needs to be gratified also gradually and increasingly diminishes. Under such emotional deprivation, especially if prolonged, many elderly become preoccupied with suspicions, imaginations, or fantasies, while others act out their needs impulsively or in a perverted manner. The ultimate outcome is either severe depression or disintegration of the personality with the emergence of psychotic symptoms such as delusions and hallucinations. This explains why the clinical manifestation of dementia sometimes can be severe in the presence of only mild to moderate structural brain impairment. These psychiatric disorders may also aggravate the already declining physical health and hence lead to a vicious cycle of progressive deterioration.

DEPRESSION.   Depression is common among the aged, the most common underlying psychogenic factor being a lowering of self-esteem. It may result from declining health; from social isolation and lack of emotional gratification; or from loss of prestige, social position, and economic status brought on after involuntary retirement. The emphasis on the value of productiveness and the general attitude toward old persons in our society undoubtedly add further insult to the already lowered self-esteem of old persons.

The differential diagnosis between affective disorder and dementia has long been emphasized because the former generally is more amenable to treatment. Nonetheless, depression in senescence is frequently overlooked, largely because it does not always follow the same clinical picture as depression in younger patients. In the depression of later life, the manifestations of depressive mood such as sad or guilty feelings, self-deprecatory thoughts, and crying spells are frequently inconspicuous, while psychomotor retardation, impairment of attention and memory, somatic symptoms, and loss of libido and initiative are more prominent. Many of these manifestations can easily be mistakenly attributed to an organic origin. Occasionally, the psychomotor retardation and regression are so severe that of themselves they may simulate dementia. More often, however, dementia and depression occur simultaneously in the same individual. The differentiation of the two components is difficult, if not impossible, and at times only a therapeutic trial with antidepressant or electroconvulsive treatment clarifies the situation. With treatment a patient may improve enough to make a reasonably good adjustment in the community in spite of the persistence of dementia or brain impairment.

Social Factors

Mental disorders in aged persons, like those in the general population, relate to many social factors. It is unclear, however, how directly these factors contribute to the development of dementia in old age since many are likely the outcome rather than the cause. They are important, nonetheless, since their presence often complicates and aggravates the clinical picture or the natural course of dementia, and some of them are readily prevented or corrected.

Social factors or conditions that have been considered as significantly associated with mental disorders of old age include: sex, cultural background, marital status, education, employment, income, family organization, living arrangements, condition and location of dwelling, type of household, and social outlets. [5,22] The common denominator for most of these social variables is the socioeconomic status of the elderly. For almost all elderly, aging means, sooner or later, loss of employment, spouse, relatives, and friends as well as decline in physical health, mental ability, income, prestige, and standard of living. All these may lead to a lowering of self-esteem and morale. Old persons of low socioeconomic status have more physical illness than those with high status. This is, to a great extent, the outcome of inadequate housing, nutrition, and medical care — all commonly asociated with poverty. The elderly individual of low socioeconomic status has less contact with relatives or friends and is less active in various social or organizational activities than elderly individuals of high socioeconomic status. The outcome of such lack of social involvement is usually emotional deprivation and an enhancement of the declining physical health and self-esteem. Low socioeconomic status thus frequently predisposes to an early onset and a rapid development of intellectual deterioration. The relationship between dementia and poverty is particularly obvious among institutionalized elderly persons.

Another important factor is environmental stress. The ability of an individual to cope with these stresses is usually reduced in old age, particularly when there is significant psychomotor retardation and impairment of memory. Because of their difficulties in understanding and remembering new experiences, elderly persons are extremely sensitive to change in their environment. Not infrequently a minor change in the household or in family relationships may precipitate a severe psychological reaction.

CONCLUSION — DEMENTIA AS A SOCIO-PSYCHO-SOMATIC DISORDER

Old age is associated with many changes. There is usually a decline in physical health and such intellectual abilities as memory, learning, and perception. There is very often also a loss of prestige, income, and social status. How well a person can adjust in his old age in a given environment depends to a great extent on how successfully he can cope with these changes as well as with various stresses from his environment.

The intellectual deterioration commonly seen among aged persons undoubtedly is closely related to the structural and functional impairment of the brain, which may or may not be recognized by the clinical and laboratory methods currently available. With a given brain impairment some individuals follow a pattern of simple and gradual intellectual deterioration and are without any significant complication. They are able to maintain a relatively active life and make a reasonably good adjustment in the community. In contrast, many others deteriorate rapidly and present a variety of complications —depression, regression, agitation, paranoid symptoms. The differences between these two groups are very likely the result of the differences in their

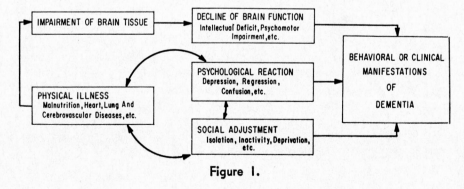

Figure I.

physical health, socioeconomic status, environment, and personality—that is, their emotional needs, self-expectations, and defense mechanisms.

Dementia as a clinical syndrome can therefore be viewed as a socio-psycho-somatic disorder (Fig. 1). Although brain impairment is the obligatory factor in most, if not all, cases of intellectual deterioration, many socio-psychological factors also play an important contributory or complicating role. These socio-psychological factors may aggravate the behavioral manifestations of intellectual deterioration. They may also accelerate the decline of physical health, which, in turn, may affect the brain as well as the socio-psychological condition of the individual. Frequently, all these factors interact with each other and form a vicious cycle that leads to further deterioration. Since little can be done about brain tissue that has lost its functional capacity, the interaction of these social, psychological, and somatic factors often becomes the most important determinant of the course and outcome of patients with dementia. Early recognition and correction of these factors may help prevent the development of complications and slow the progression of deterioration.

REFERENCES

1. Arab, A.: *Plaques séniles et artériosclerose cérébrale.* Rev. Neurol. 91: 22-36, 1954.

2. Birren, J. E.: Increments and decrements in the intellectual status of the aged, in Simon, A., and Epstein, L. J. (eds.) : *Aging in Modern Society: Psychiatric Research Report 23.* American Psychiatric Association, Washington, D. C., 1968, pp. 207-214.

3. Blessed, G., Tomlinson, B. E., and Roth, M.: *The association between quantitative measures of dementia and of senile change in the cerebral grey matter of elderly subjects.* Brit. J. Psychiat. 114:797-811, 1968.

4. Botwinick, J.: *Cognitive Processes in Maturity and Old Age.* Springer Publishing Co., Inc., New York, 1967.

5. Busse, E. W.: Brain syndromes associated with disturbances in metabolism, growth, and nutrition, in Freedman, A. M., and Kaplan, H. I. (eds.) : *Comprehensive Textbook of Psychiatry.* The Williams & Wilkins Co., Baltimore, 1967, pp, 726-740.

6. Busse, E. W., and Wang, H. S.: *The value of electroencephalography in geriatrics.* Geriatrics 20:906-924, 1965.

7. Butler, R. N., Dastur, D. K., and Perlin, S.: *Relationship of senile manifestations and chronic brain syndromes to cerebral circulation and metabolism.* J. Psychiat. Res. 3:229-238, 1965.

8. Confrey, E. A., and Goldstein, M. S.: The health status of aging people, in Tibbitts, C. (ed.) : *Handbook of Social Gerontology.* University of Chicago Press, Chicago, 1960, pp. 165-207.

9. Corsellis, J. A. N.: *Mental Illness and the Ageing Brain.* Oxford University Press, London, 1962.

10. DASTUR, D. K., LANE, M. H., HANSEN, D. B., KETY, S. S., PERLIN, S., BUTLER, R. N., AND SOKOLOFF, L.: Effects of aging on cerebral circulation and metabolism in man, in Birren, J. E., Butler, R. N., Greenhouse, S. W., Sokoloff, L., and Yarrow, M. R. (eds.) : *Human Aging: A Biological Behavioral Study.* U. S. Government Printing Office, Washington, D. C., 1963, pp. 59-76.

11. EISDORFER, C.: *Psychologic reaction to cardiovascular change in the aged.* Mayo Clin. Proc. 42:620-636, 1967.

12. EISDORFER, C.: *The WAIS performance of the aged: A retest evaluation.* J. Gerontol. 18:169-172, 1963.

13. HALSTEAD, W. C.: Biological intelligence and differential aging, in Webber, I. L. (ed.) : *Aging: A Current Appraisal.* University of Florida Press, Gainesville, 1956, pp. 63-75.

14. JARVIK, L. F., KALLMAN, F. J., AND FALEK, A.: *Intellectual changes in aged twins.* J. Gerontol. 17:289-294, 1962.

15. KATZ, L., NEAL, M. W., AND SIMON, A.: Observations on psychic mechanisms in organic psychoses of the aged, in Hock, P. H., and Zubin, J. (eds.) : *Psychopathology of Aging.* Grune & Stratton, Inc., New York, 1961, pp. 160-181.

16. KIEV, A., CHAPMAN, L. F., GUTHRIE, T. C., AND WOLFF, H. G.: *The highest integrative functions and diffuse cerebral atrophy.* Neurology 12: 385-393, 1962.

17. OAKLEY, D. P.: *Senile dementia, some aetiological factors.* Brit. J. Psychiat. 111:414-419, 1965.

18. OBRIST, W. D., AND BISSELL, L. F.: *The electroencephalogram of aged patients with cardiac and cerebral vascular disease.* J. Gerontol. 10:315-330, 1955.

19. OBRIST, W. D., CHIVIAN, E., CRONQVIST, S., AND INGVAR, D. H.: *Regional cerebral blood flow in senile and presenile dementia.* Neurology. 20:315-322, 1970.

20. OBRIST, W. D., AND HENRY, C. E.: *Electroencephalographic findings in aged psychiatric patients.* J. Nerv. Ment. Dis. 126:254-267, 1958.

21. PIERCE, R. C., AND BERKMAN, P. L.: Change in intellectual functioning, in Lowenthal, M. F., Berkman, P. L., and Associates (eds.) : *Aging and Mental Disorder in San Francisco.* Jossey-Bass, Inc., Publishers, San Francisco, 1967, pp. 177-189.

22. RILEY, M. W., AND FONER, A.: *Aging and Society. I. An Inventory of Research Findings.* Russell Sage Foundation, New York, 1968.

23. ROTHSCHILD, D.: *Pathologic changes in senile psychoses and their psychobiologic significance.* Amer. J. Psychiat. 93:757-785, 1937.

24. SOKOLOFF, L.: Circulation and metabolism of brain in relation to the process of aging, in Birren, J. E., Imus, H. A., and Windle, W. F. (eds.) : *The Process of Aging in the Nervous System.* Charles C Thomas, Publisher, Springfield, Ill., 1959, pp. 113-126.

161

25. TOMLINSON, B. E.: Personal communication quoted in Reference No. 3 above, 1966.

26. TOMLINSON, B. E., BLESSED, G., AND ROTH, M.: *Observations on the brain of non-demented old people.* J. Neurol. Sci. 7:331-356, 1968.

27. TRIER, T. R.: *Characteristics of mentally ill aged: A comparison of patients with psychogenic disorders and patients with organic brain syndromes.* J. Gerontol. 21:354-364, 1966.

28. WANG, H. S.: *The brain and intellectual function in senescence.* American Psychological Association Meeting, San Francisco, California, 1968.

29. WANG, H. S.: Organic brain syndromes, in Busse, E. W., and Pfeiffer, E. (eds.): *Behavior and Adaptation in Late Life.* Little, Brown, and Company, Boston, 1969, pp. 263-287.

30. WANG, H. S., AND BUSSE, E. W.: *EEG of healthy old persons, a longitudinal study. I. Dominant background activity and occipital rhythm.* J. Gerontol. 24:419-426, 1969.

31. WANG, H. S., OBRIST, W. D., AND BUSSE, E. W.: *Neurophysiological correlates of the intellectual function of elderly persons living in the community.* Amer. J. Psychiat. 126:1205-1212, 1970.

32. WECHSLER, D.: *The Measurement and Appraisal of Adult Intelligence,* ed. 4. The Williams & Wilkins Co., Baltimore, 1958.

33. WILLANGER, R., THYGESEN, P., NIELSEN, R., AND PETERSEN, O.: *Intellectual impairment and cerebral atrophy—a psychological, neurological and radiological investigation.* Danish Med. Bull. 15:65-93, 1968.

Chapter 10

Diseases Presenting as Dementia

Gunter R. Haase, M.D.

Many diseases may be accompanied by progressive reduction of intellectual function. In some it may be the initial clinical feature, in others appearing long after more definitive and specific physiological changes have occurred. The conditions discussed in this chapter all can cause dementia and in many dementia may be the initial or leading manifestation. The most important of these conditions are listed in Table 1. Beginning with the section on Metabolic Disorders are listed disorders in which the dementia may be brought about by reduced supply of oxygen or other nutrients to the central nervous system, by the cerebral damage brought about by trauma or infectious agents, by alterations in the intracranial pressure relationships, or by exogenous or endogenous toxic substances. An important part of the investigation of the patient with

Table 1. Diseases causing dementia

Diffuse Parenchymatous Diseases of the Central Nervous System	**Normal pressure hydrocephalus**
So-called presenile dementias	**Deficiency diseases**
Alzheimer's disease	Wernicke-Korsakoff syndrome
Pick's disease	Pellagra
Creutzfeldt-Jakob disease	Marchiafava-Bignami disease
Kraepelin's disease	Vitamin B_{12} deficiency
Parkinson-dementia complex of Guam	
Huntington's chorea	**Toxins and drugs**
	Metals
Senile dementia	Organic compounds
	Carbon monoxide
Other degenerative diseases	Drugs
Hallervorden-Spatz disease	
Spinocerebellar degenerations	**Brain tumors**
Progressive myoclonus epilepsy	
Progressive supranuclear palsy	**Trauma**
Parkinson's disease	Open and closed head injuries
	Punch-drunk syndrome
Metabolic disorders	Subdural hematoma
Myxedema	Heat stroke
Disorders of the parathyroid glands	
Wilson's disease	**Infections**
Liver disease	Brain abscess
Hypoglycemia	Bacterial meningitis
Remote effects of carcinoma	Fungal meningitis
Cushing's syndrome	Encephalitis
Uremia	Progressive multifocal leukoencephalopathy
	Behçet's syndrome
Vascular disorders	Kuru
Arteriosclerosis	Lues
Inflammatory disease of blood vessels	
Aortic arch syndrome	**Other**
Binswanger's disease	Multiple sclerosis
Arteriovenous malformations	Muscular dystrophies
	Whipple's disease
Hypoxia and anoxia	Concentration-camp syndrome

decompensation of intellectual functions is the exclusion of these possible causes, since the process in some instances may be amenable to treatment. There remains a group of disorders in which—at least at the present position of medical knowledge—the disease process is one affecting primarily the cells of the nervous system (Diffuse Parenchymatous Diseases of the Central Nervous System, Table 1). The chapter will concern itself mainly with these diseases.

DIFFUSE PARENCHYMATOUS DISEASES OF THE CENTRAL NERVOUS SYSTEM

So-called Presenile Dementias

Alzheimer's Disease and Pick's Disease

Alzheimer's disease and Pick's disease, while pathologically distinct, resemble each other so closely in their clinical manifestations that their discussion under a common heading appears justified. Criteria to separate these diseases on clinical grounds[200, 203, 212, 241, 256] are not universally accepted, and the possibility of a separation on the basis of clinical or neuroradiological features is denied or described as extremely difficult by some writers on the subject.[10, 147, 157]

Both diseases begin usually between the ages of 45 and 60 years. Instances with onset in early adult life have been recorded,[138] and at the upper age range the delimitation from the so-called senile dementia is blurred.

The preceding history, both with regard to physical and emotional health, is usually unremarkable in the persons afflicted. The sexes are approximately equally affected, although in some reports, females are said to be more susceptible to both disorders.[84, 138, 243] Familial occurrence has been described in both diseases. In a few families with Alzheimer's disease, inheritance as a dominant trait has been suggested,[61, 101, 178] while in other instances a multifactorial inheritance has been considered more likely.[203]

In Pick's disease, familial instances suggest a dominant autosomal mode of inheritance.[178, 203]

The incidence of Alzheimer's disease in most studies is considerably greater than that of Pick's disease, although in Sjögren's study,[203] both occurred with the same frequency.

While the loss of intellectual functions is the hallmark of both disorders, the initial symptoms may suggest a psychogenic illness by such features as anxiety, depression, restlessness, or sleep disorder, or, less commonly, by hallucinations, particularly of a visual nature. Pronounced jealousy was the first evidence of the disease in Alzheimer's original patient,[12] and paranoid traits have been prominent in other instances. Disturbances of memory may soon follow these initial deviations, or may be the first manifestation of disorder. In either case,

165

impairment of intellectual function soon dominates the clinical picture and may be accompanied by loss of spontaneity and indolence, or by purposeless overactivity. Facetiousness ("moria") is seen frequently, as is a disturbance in the formation of moral and ethical judgments. The patients commit indiscretions in their professional and social conduct; they may prove themselves incapable of handling their business and financial affairs and may run afoul of the law. Their insight is impaired, and their foresight untempered by reality.

The evolution of both disorders is marked by the steadily progressing attrition of mental capacities. While in the early stages, the gravest defect concerns memory, in particular that for recent events, eventually all intellectual functions will be affected. The rate of progression varies considerably, some patients reaching social incapacity in a few months, while in others this stage may be reached only after several years.

As the features of intellectual deterioration progress, focal manifestations of neurological disease will frequently supervene. Disorientation in space may result in the patient's becoming lost in familiar surroundings, even in his own home. Disorders of symbol utilization, such as dysphasia, dyslexia, dysgraphia, and dyspraxia, are common (see Chapter 3) and may be coupled with repetitive utterances (logoclonia) or repetitive actions. Other focal signs, such as convulsions or central facial paralysis, are common enough to be considered part of the clinical picture, while evidence of a disorder of the upper motor neuron type is usually, but not always,[101] lacking.

As the disorder develops, there may be occasional bursts of excitement, but the characteristic course is one of increasing apathy and indolence. The patients show severe dementia, failure of comprehending and communicating with their environment, and eventually incontinence. Forced grasping and groping, suck and snout reflexes, if not present since earlier stages of the disease, appear. Some patients show voracious hunger, in spite of which physical emaciation will progress. Death usually occurs from 5 to 10 years after the diagnosis of the disease, and respiratory infections are the most common cause of death.

As these two disorders have been described thus far, no notice has been taken of the alleged differences between Alzheimer's and Pick's disease. There is an extensive body of literature dealing with semeiological characteristics of either disorder. Many of these claims are based on small series of cases and have been subsequently disputed by other writers. Other claims are of a statistical nature, asserting, for instance, that convulsions occur more often in Alzheimer's disease, or that localizing signs are "not very evident" in Alzheimer's disease and "more evident" in Pick's disease.[256]

The clinician confronted with a patient with dementia in middle life will not find much assistance from such indicators. Perhaps more serious consideration must be given to the claim[203] that patients with Alzheimer's disease will, either early or in the later stages of their illness, show a "rigidity of extrapyramidal type" with cogwheel phenomenon. Coupled with this is said to be a syndrome of "direct forward staring." This syndrome, observed in one series[203] in 14 of 23 patients with Alzheimer's disease, consists of a failure to move the eyes in either plane ("the gaze is as if it were locked in a fixed forward stare"). Spatial disorientation may be one of the chief symptoms of Alzheimer's disease.[54]

The increase in muscle tone, referred to above, was found in one study in 14 of 18 patients with Alzheimer's disease[203] and was not accompanied by tremor. Myoclonic jerks have, however, been encountered in some cases.[61,101] Sjögren[203] observed the frequent occurrence of a disorder of gait in patients with Alzheimer's disease. He described the difficulty experienced by patients in the earlier stages of this disease as one in "realizing the rhythm and coordinating of the movements necessary for normal gait . . . the gait is slow, unsteady, clumsy, but without pulsion phenomenon." Sjögren, Sjögren, and Lindgren[203] believed the disturbance resembled apraxia of gait, and suggested that this disorder of gait may be ascribed to lesions in the prefrontal regions. At a later time in the evolution of the disorder, some patients may demonstrate "marche à petits pas."

The disturbance of gait observed in patients with Alzheimer's disease was not seen in any of the patients with Pick's disease. The incidence of changes of muscular tone was also significantly greater in the Alzheimer disease cases than in those with Pick's disease, being present in 14 patients with Alzheimer's disease and in 1 case with Pick's disease.

The occurrence of convulsive seizures has been deemed another feature enabling the clinician to differentiate Alzheimer's disease from Pick's disease. In Sjögren's study, convulsions occurred in 4 out of 18 patients with histologically proved Alzheimer's disease and in 1 of 18 patients with histologically proved Pick's disease.

A number of other features asserted to be of distinguishing value, such as the presence or absence of motor excitement or apathy, occurred with sufficient frequency in both groups to put their differential-diagnostic value into question.

In summary, it is very difficult on clinical grounds alone to attempt a differentiation of Alzheimer's disease from Pick's disease. At present, judgment must be reserved about the weight added to the diagnosis of Alzheimer's disease by the presence of extrapyramidal features and of the gait disturbance described above.

The EEG does not show specific abnormalities relating to the subgroups of dementia, but the incidence of abnormalities is reported to be greater and more consistent in Alzheimer's disease than in any of the other entities.[86,127,129] Absence or reduction of alpha activity is particularly striking in patients with Alzheimer's disease and may progress to the emergence of patterns in the theta and delta range, at times occurring in bursts. In Pick's disease, the EEG may be normal.[86,223] The degree of EEG abnormality does not appear to be related to the degree of cerebral atrophy or the duration of the illness. It has been asserted that in Alzheimer's disease the severe degrees of EEG abnormality tend to be correlated with severe degrees of dementia.[86]

The cerebrospinal fluid in both conditions described is usually normal.

Pneumoencephalographic investigation will usually demonstrate cerebral atrophy by increase in the width of the sulcal markings and by ventricular enlargement, particularly of the anterior and temporal horns, but will not assist in the differential diagnosis between Pick's and Alzheimer's disease.[203,228]

Other laboratory studies are of little value in the differential diagnosis, except for their use in excluding other diseases, such as syphilis of the central nervous system.

It is possible sometimes to establish the diagnosis during life by cortical biopsy.[87] More commonly, the autopsy findings provide the conclusive evidence. In both disorders, specific pathological changes are restricted to the brain and will impress, on gross inspection, by the evidence of cortical atrophy, combined with ventricular enlargement. The brain weight is reduced, often below 1000 gm. In Alzheimer's disease, the atrophy is diffuse over the cortical mantle, but most striking in the frontal and occipital lobes. In Pick's disease, the atrophy is most impressive in the frontal and temporal lobes. In the temporal lobes, the atrophy usually involves the middle and inferior temporal gyri, and characteristically, the superior temporal gyrus is involved only in its anterior third. The subcortical white matter participates in the shrinkage of the affected areas and this has led to the term *lobar sclerosis*. Subcortical gray structures may also participate in the atrophy.[138,258]

Histologically, Alzheimer's disease is characterized by neurofibrillary degenerative changes in the neurons and by the presence of argyrophilic plaques, primarily in the cerebral cortex, and less consistently in the basal ganglia. These findings are accompanied by a loss of nerve cells. In Pick's disease, the prominent histological abnormality is a cell loss in the affected areas, associated with extensive gliosis. The cell loss is most impressive in the outer layers of the cortex. The remaining nerve cells may show swelling and argyrophilic inclusions ("Pick cells"). Cases showing histological features of both Alzheimer's and Pick's disease have been described.[25]

Electron microscopic studies[120,134,229,230] have shown the neurofibrillary alteration to consist of hollow fibrils, which displace the normal organelles of the cells. The plaques have a core of amyloid fibrils, surrounded by abnormal dendrites and axons. It is probable that microglial cells are the source of the amyloid material.

Creutzfeldt-Jakob Disease

Creutzfeldt-Jakob disease is a diffuse disorder of the nervous system, marked by neuronal degeneration, glial proliferation, and, frequently, status spongiosus.

Not only the nomenclature, but also the clinical range of its manifestations, has been a matter of dispute. Although a term such as *subacute presenile polioencephalopathy*[32] may be a more adequate description of the entity, the eponymic term is sufficiently honored by usage to make its displacement unlikely.

The first report, published by Creutzfeldt in 1920,[42] concerned a 23-year-old woman, who died after a neurological illness of $2\frac{1}{2}$ years' duration. Pathological examination of the brain disclosed diffuse alterations in the gray matter of the cerebral cortex and of subcortical gray structures. In the following year, Jakob reported three similar cases, to which he added two more instances in his monograph[110] on the extrapyramidal disorders, published in 1923.

About 200 cases have been reported up to the present, the majority having been confirmed by histological study (biopsy or postmortem examination).[145] Familial incidence has been noted in three families, with dominant autosomal transmission the apparent mode of inheritance.[146]

The disease usually becomes apparent between the ages of 40 and 60 years, and the sexes are equally affected. While some afflicted persons have lived for several years after the diagnosis, the usual duration is measured in months. About half of all patients survived less than 9 months.[145]

In the early stages, neurotic manifestations, such as anxiety, nervousness, excessive startle reaction, fatigability, depression and loss of appetite may predominate, while in other instances, loss of memory, euphoria, confusion, lability in the affective sphere, hallucinations, delusions or behavioral changes suggest a functional psychotic disorder. In still other patients, the illness may declare itself from the outset as a neurological disorder, by disturbances of speech or coordination, or by paresthesiae, visual disturbances, involuntary movements, or episodic loss of consciousness. Transient remission of symptoms, lasting weeks to months, may occur, but in most instances, the range of symptoms increases, and definite signs of neurological disease appear, often asymmetrically. Most consistently, these indicate involvement of the upper motor neuron, with appearance of suck and snout responses, forced grasping, plantar extensor responses and spasticity, or manifestations of extrapyramidal disease, including tremors, choreiform or athetoid movements, myoclonic discharges, dystonia, or muscular rigidity.

Signs indicating disorder of the lower motor neuron, such as muscular wasting and fasciculations, and signs of brainstem involvement, such as diplopia, anisocoria, or nystagmus, appear with less regularity. Cerebellar dysfunction may be the initial manifestation or may appear at a later stage in the course of the disease.[32] An exaggerated startle response is a common observation in this disorder,[63] and convulsive seizures have been observed.

As the illness progresses, the patient may become mute and assume

169

decorticate or decerebrate postures. Some patients lapse into an akinetic mute state or coma, which usually is fatally terminated by a respiratory infection.

In the majority of instances, examination of the spinal fluid will yield normal results,[198] although increase of the protein content, usually of a mild degree, has been reported in about 10 per cent of cases.

The pneumoencephalogram usually shows evidence of mild to moderate ventricular enlargement and cortical atrophy, particularly over the frontal portions of the brain.[145] Abnormalities of the EEG have been reported to occur in more than 90 per cent of the patients.[145] In the early stages, diffuse or focal slowing may be observed. As the disorder progresses, slow spikes and spike-wave complexes may be superimposed on a slow, low-voltage background activity. These slow bursts may be accompanied by myoclonic jerking. Considered pathognomonic by some,[63] this pattern has also been found in instances of subacute inclusion body encephalitis[126] and has not been invariably present in the reported cases of Creutzfeldt-Jakob disease.

On pathological examination, mild to moderate atrophic changes are observed in the cortex, at times predominantly in the frontal, parietal or temporal areas. With less consistency, pathological alterations are seen in the basal ganglia, corticospinal tracts, motor neurons, thalamus and cerebellum.

Histologically, diffuse ganglion cell loss is observed in the affected areas, while the remaining cells may be swollen with lipochrome. Status spongiosus, particularly of the deeper cortical layers, is a common finding, as is astrocytic proliferation. Electron microscopic studies[83,142] have shown the "status spongiosus" to be due to dilatation of cellular processes, involving astrocytes and neurons.

The etiology of the condition is unknown. The possibility of a relationship to pellagra of the central nervous system has been commented upon.[138] Both astrocytes and neurons have been considered to be the cellular elements primarily affected by the disorder.[67,193,198] Experimental transmission of the disease by inoculation of brain biopsy material from an affected patient into a chimpanzee has been done.[78] Thirteen months later, the animal developed a subacute progressive brain disease, with clinical course and neuropathological findings "remarkably similar" to those in the human patient, suggesting that the disease is caused by a transmissible agent, probably a virus. Viruslike particles have been found in brain biopsies from patients with Creutzfeldt-Jakob disease.[244]

The protean clinical and pathological manifestations of this disorder have resulted in considerable controversy, and it has been suggested that the cases falling into this group may be heterogeneous. This has resulted in attempts to classify subtypes, or to separate altogether groups of patients on the basis of clinical or pathological characteristics.[145] Although, at present, judgment must be reserved about the validity of establishing subtypes, certain groups of cases are sufficiently different from the majority to warrant consideration:

1. Nevin and associates[158] presented eight patients with clinical features similar to the ones described above. These authors felt, however, that the pathological features of their cases, and of 15 others collected from the literature, differed from the "classical" Creutzfeldt-Jakob disease, insofar as status spongiosus was a more common feature of an entity they termed *subacute spongiform encephalopathy* (SSE), with a predeliction for the occipital cortex, little or no degeneration of the motor nuclei in brainstem and spinal cord, or degeneration of myelinated tracts. The type of cell shrinkage, as well as the behavior of astrocytes, also was, in their opinion, different from the findings in Creutzfeldt-Jakob disease.

Nevin and his group[158] included under the heading of SSE two of the patients originally described by Heidenhain.[99] To these cases, and one of their own, Meyer, Leigh, and Bagg[151] attached the designation of *Heidenhain's syndrome*. Clinically, these cases were characterized by cortical blindness and dementia, and pathologically by involvement of the occipital cortex. Nevin's group believed that vascular impairment was the most likely cause of SSE. The validity of separating these cases has been contested.[198]

2. Patients with prominent thalamic involvement were reported by Stern,[213] Schulman,[195] and Garcin, Brion, and Khochnevis.[75]

3. An ataxic form, with prominent involvement of the granular layer of the cerebellum, has been recorded by Brownell and Oppenheimer,[32] who, in addition to four cases of their own, collected six similar instances from the literature.

McMenemey[138] suggests that at the present time it appears most reasonable to consider these conditions as constituting "a group of disorders of like character," without necessarily implying the same etiology for all cases.

Kraepelin's Disease

Another form of dementia, characterized by catatonia, was described by Kraepelin in 1910. McMenemey[138] states that 17 cases have been reported. Other features included anxiety, depression, restlessness, and speech defects. The usual duration of the illness was 1 to 2 years. Pathological changes included destruction of the Nissl substance in the neurons, particularly in the frontal and central areas and in Ammon's horn, and eventual loss of ganglion cells. Schaumburg and Suzuki,[193] relating a form of presenile dementia in six members of a family, observed pathological changes similar to those described in Kraepelin's disease, including atrophy of all lobes of the brain, with diffuse loss of neurons in all layers, only slight glial proliferation, and diffuse demyelination in the white matter. No specific changes, such as neurofibrillary degeneration or senile plaques, were observed. Schaumburg and Suzuki[193] felt that in the majority of cases reported as Kraepelin's disease, other plausible causes could explain the pathological changes, and they agreed with McMenemey[138] that the existence of Kraepelin's disease as a pathological

171

entity is doubtful. Disregarding arguments about nomenclature, their paper brings to attention other, nonspecific types of dementia in adult life. The pedigree presented by Schaumburg and Suzuki suggests a dominant pattern of inheritance.

Parkinson-Dementia Complex of Guam

Among the indigenous Chamorro population of Guam and neighboring islands, a high incidence of neurological disease has been found.[56,57,104–106,141,181] While a syndrome resembling amyotrophic lateral sclerosis (ALS) is the most common neurological illness, accounting for approximately 10 per cent of all deaths in Guam, frequent instances were observed of a disorder combining progressive dementia with features of Parkinson's disease, and at times with features of amyotrophic lateral sclerosis.[104,106] Subsequent studies suggest that in the Mariana and Caroline Islands persons of ethnic background other than the Chamorros may also fall victim to this disorder.[56]

A reevaluation of these disorders in 1966[56] concerned 176 patients, of whom 104 presented clinically as ALS, while 72 presented with the Parkinson-dementia complex. One half of 22 additional patients, initially observed to be suffering from Parkinson's disease without dementia, developed features of dementia within a year of onset of the illness.

Those individuals presenting with ALS were usually between 40 and 50 years of age (age range 20 to 67 years), while the patients first afflicted with the Parkinson-dementia complex were usually in their 50's. Of the 104 ALS patients, 5 developed the Parkinson-dementia syndrome (on the average 5 years after onset of the ALS): 5 patients developed Parkinson's disease without dementia; and 2 patients, an "organic mental syndrome" without parkinsonian features. Of the original 72 Parkinson-dementia patients, 27 developed ALS.

The presenting signs of the dementia were usually memory deficits and disorientation for time, place, and person, associated with or followed by changes in personality or behavior patterns, which progressed to increasing confusion and apathy. Bradykinesia, rigidity, and tremor completed the picture in the typical case.

Neuropathological studies showed that all 48 ALS patients examined histologically had, in addition to the characteristics of ALS, the features of Parkinson-dementia, and of 45 patients with Parkinson-dementia, 17 had the histological features of ALS.

The pathological characteristics of the Parkinson-dementia complex were diffuse cerebral atrophy, particularly of the frontal and temporal lobes, with ventricular enlargement ranging from minimal to severe. The globus pallidus and substantia nigra were atrophied, and in the latter area there was loss of the normal pigment. Widespread neurofibrillary changes were seen in the cortex and subcortical nuclei, while senile (argyrophilic) plaques and Lewy bodies were rarely encountered.[105]

The presence of similar neuropathological changes in the Guam cases of ALS, as well as the clinical association of ALS and Parkinson-dementia complex, may be considered as evidence that these cases share a common etiological factor, whose nature thus far has remained elusive. The evidence is not sufficiently strong to point to a genetically determined basis, and the geographical grouping of cases still leaves open the possibility of environmental factors.[181]

Huntington's Chorea

George Huntington[108] described in 1872 a disorder affecting a mother and daughter, characterized by choreiform movements and progressive mental deterioration. Similar patients had been described earlier,[178] and subsequent reports indicated the disease to occur in almost all races. The sexes are equally affected.

Various genetic studies[178] are in agreement about the dominant inheritance of the disease. Clinical manifestations usually do not become apparent until the fourth or fifth decade of life, and there is at present no means available to identify persons destined to develop the disease at an earlier age, save perhaps the EEG, which is reported to "possibly become abnormal a few years before clinical signs are present,"[124,170] and psychological tests.[85]

Cases with onset earlier than described above are on record,[113,143] and in other instances, the onset may be delayed until old age. Frequently, the exact onset is difficult to determine, since family members may report that the afflicted person appeared "nervous," "fidgety," or mentally unstable for many years.

Usually the disease becomes manifest by the appearance of the choreic movements, affecting facial expression, or the muscles of the trunk or extremities. While at first the afflicted person may be able to incorporate the involuntary movements into purposeful actions, he gradually loses this measure of control; his voluntary activities, and even his repose, become disrupted by continual movements. They may interfere with his ability to fall asleep, although, once asleep, they will cease. Respiration and speech, as well as gait and stance, are affected by the movements.

Usually, mental alterations will become evident after the appearance of involuntary movements, while in other instances, they will develop simultaneously or even precede the movement disorder. They may become apparent as neurotic manifestations, such as anxiety states, irritability or depression, or as simple deterioration of intellectual capacities, such as memory loss, impairment of abstract reasoning, or failure to grasp simple concepts. Still other patients show faulty judgments in professional or financial matters, or become offensive because of moral or ethical lapses. At times, paranoid or delusional features suggesting a "functional" psychosis may predominate. The incidence of suicide is high in families with Huntington's chorea.[147]

Some afflicted members of a family may show only the choreic features or only the dementia. In some cases, particularly those with early onset, hypokinesia and rigidity may be prominent features.[26] In a few instances, convulsive seizures have been observed.

Laboratory studies usually yield normal values, although at times the protein level of the cerebrospinal fluid is raised. The pneumoencephalogram may show enlargment of the ventricles, with loss of convexity of the caudate nucleus, and evidence of cortical atrophy, but the severity of atrophy does not closely parallel the clinical manifestations.[28]

Claims that the intracellular level of magnesium and calcium is elevated in Huntington's chorea[116] were not confirmed in later studies.[33,97]

The progression of the disorder is a slow one, and the average survival after onset is approximately 15 years, respiratory infections being the most common cause of death.

Pathological alterations specific for the disease are restricted to the nervous system and consist of loss of nerve cells in the caudate nucleus and putamen and in the deeper layers of the cortex, particularly in the frontal lobes. Slight to marked glial proliferation may be observed in the affected areas of the basal ganglia.[138]

Senile Dementia

The clinical picture of senile dementia is similar to that of Alzheimer's disease, although, by definition, the onset is later in life, and the progression is slower. Defects of memory are usually observed early, followed by confusion in space and time, inconsistency in work habits, reduction of attention and interest, and deterioration in personal habits. The patients may misplace objects, and then accuse others of theft. They frequently will roam at night, wander away from home, or, in the hospital, enter other patients' rooms. They may become incontinent or satisfy their toilet needs in inappropriate places. At times, the onset of the illness is related by family members to an acute emotional or physical stress, such as an infection or operation. Characteristics already discernible in the premorbid personality may become accentuated, while in other instances, witnesses assert that the changes in the patient bear no relation to his previous personality.

Subtypes have been described,[53] although the lines of distinction are rarely sharply drawn in the individual patient: (1) simple deterioration, (2) depressed and agitated type, (3) delirious and confused type, (4) hyperactive type with motor restlessness and loquaciousness, (5) paranoid type.

Focal neurological signs are not part of the picture, although muscular rigidity, gait disturbances, and tremor may be observed.

Physicians with appropriate experience will recognize a certain arbitrariness in the classification described, since individual patients may not only show the features of more than one type but may also be classified differently at different points in the evolution of their disorder. The most constant feature is the progressive attrition of memory and other intellectual capacities, although not only the age of onset but also the rate of progression may vary greatly. While the disease is not fatal in itself, it will at times be responsible for accidents or exposure and in other instances indirectly result in bedsores or systemic infection.

Close relatives of patients with senile dementia have a risk four times that of the general population of developing the disease, and either a multifactorial or a dominant mode of inheritance is likely.[178]

The pathological substrate in senile dementia, in particular its relation to the changes of Alzheimer's disease, has been a matter of controversy and has been summarized by McMenemey.[137,138]

The brains of most patients with senile dementia show diffuse atrophy, argyrophilic plaques, and Alzheimer's neurofibrillary changes. "If one accepts them, in spite of their late age of onset, as instances of Alzheimer's disease, then few cases remain to be labelled senile dementia."[138] Neumann and Cohn[157] and Raskin and Ehrenberg[180] also believe that no sound argument can be advanced for separating the cases of presenile dementia of Alzheimer type from cases of identical clinical and pathological features but a later onset. A direct relationship between the number of plaques in cerebral gray matter and the degree of dementia has been observed.[27]

There remain a number of instances of senile brain disease in which neither significant Alzheimer changes nor evidence of other disease, such as arteriosclerosis or infectious processes, are observed. For these, the term *simple senile atrophy* (atrophia senilis simplex) has been recommended.[138]

Other Degenerative Diseases

Hallervorden-Spatz Disease

Hallervorden and Spatz[94] described in 1922 a family in which 5 out of 9 siblings suffered from a disorder characterized by progressive dementia, spastic paralysis, and athetosis. The disease usually began late in the first decade of life, and progressed to death in the second or third decade. Approximately 30 verified cases have been recorded,[150] although other cases in the literature may well belong to this group.[48] Other clinical features, less constant, include foot deformities, chorea or athetosis, optic atrophy, retinitis pigmentosa, ocular palsies, dysarthria, and convulsions. Familial occurrence has been observed in some of the recorded cases.[178]

On pathological examination, rust-brown coloring has been observed in the globus pallidus and substantia nigra, due to the presence of iron-containing pigment. Associated with this have been variable degrees of cellular loss and glial proliferation and inconstant histological changes in other parts of the brain and spinal cord.

175

Spinocerebellar Degenerations

Loss of intellectual functions is observed at times in the spinocerebellar degenerations. Greenfield[88] quotes Bell and Carmichael as having found "mental deficiency" in 23 per cent of 242 families with Friedreich's ataxia. In 76 families with spastic paraplegia, the incidence was 27.5 per cent. In some instances, the intellectual changes affected only nonataxic members. Sjögren[202] observed oligophrenia in 15 of 84 cases of Friedreich's ataxia and progressive dementia in 58 per cent. Mental changes, with varying degrees of prominence, have been noted in many of the subforms of the spinocerebellar degenerations.[6,37,80,140,169]

Progressive Myoclonus Epilepsy

The familial occurrence of a disorder combining myoclonic jerking and generalized convulsions was first described by Unverricht[238] in 1891. In 1895, he added another family with a similar disorder.[239] In both families, the affected members developed myoclonic muscle contractions in late childhood or early adolescence. The progressive severity of the myoclonic contractions eventually interfered with ordinary activities, but dementia was not part of the clinical picture, nor was it evident in the cases of Lundborg.[133] In 1911, Lafora and Glueck[122] described the postmortem findings in a 17-year-old boy, who, in addition to myoclonus and generalized convulsions, had suffered from a rapidly progressing dementia. They found concentric inclusions in the neurons of cerebral cortex, basal ganglia, brainstem and spinal cord. Similar inclusions have been found in the heart, liver, and skeletal muscles of other patients.[96,196] Despite similar clinical features, Lafora bodies have not been found at autopsy in all instances, and the following types of myoclonus epilepsy are now recognized:[95,96]

1. Lafora body disease, with onset usually in the second decade of life, progressing to death in a few years, and accompanied by dementia.[96,111,196]

2. Myoclonus epilepsy in lipidosis (familial amaurotic idiocy)—the onset is usually earlier, progression may be more rapid or more protracted, dementia is less consistently present and may be accompanied by retinitis pigmentosa or macular degeneration.[95,186,252]

3. Myoclonus epilepsy in diseases with system degeneration, i.e., spinocerebellar degenerations with onset in the second decade or later, slow progression, usually without significant dementia, but with occasional presence of foot deformity, kyphoscoliosis, or ataxia in patients or their close relatives.[95,161]

Progressive Supranuclear Palsy

A group of patients was described in 1964[211] with a syndrome combining supranuclear paralysis of extraocular movements, particularly in the vertical plane, with dementia, dysarthria, pseudobulbar palsy, and dystonic rigidity of the neck and trunk. Signs of cerebellar and pyramidal dysfunction were less constant. The disorder usually began in the sixth decade and progressed to death in a few years.

Pathological changes included cell loss, neurofibrillary alterations, gliosis, and demyelination in various regions of the basal ganglia, brainstem, and cerebellum, while the cortex was usually normal.

Subsequent reports have pointed out the occurrence of involuntary movements and of involvement of brainstem nuclei.[29,45] A degenerative or vital etiology has been considered possible by Steele and co-workers,[211] who also commented on the resemblance of the histological features in this disorder to those seen in postencephalitic parkinsonism and to the Parkinson-dementia complex of Guam.

Parkinson's Disease

In his original description of the disease bearing his name, Parkinson stated that "the senses and intellect" remained unaffected.[167] Subsequently, instances of mental changes accompanying the various forms of Parkinson's disease have been recorded. Pollock and Hornabrook[177] observed variable degrees of dementia in all forms of Parkinson's disease, but "predominantly in those with associated arteriosclerosis." The relationship of arteriosclerosis to dementia will be considered in the section titled Vascular Disorders.

METABOLIC DISORDERS

Myxedema

Psychological alterations are common in patients with myxedema. These range from apathy, depression, and stupor to delusional psychosis and dementia.[112,159,192] Since other clinical signs of myxedema need not accompany the psychological and mental alterations, evaluation of thyroid function is an important part in the study of patients with progressive dementia. Unless treatment is instituted early, some degree of mental impairment may remain permanently.

Disorders of the Parathyroid Glands

In hyperparathyroidism, neurological changes are uncommon, although lethargy and confusional states may accompany hypercalcemia of any cause.[21,125] In one series of 33 cases of hyperparathyroidism, 4 patients had psychiatric manifestations.[115] Dementia, while rare, has been observed.

Neurological abnormalities are more commonly seen in patients with hypoparathyroidism and include convulsions, papilledema, paresthesia, hyperreflexia, tetany, weakness, and EEG abnormalities. Psychiatric alterations include toxic-delirious states, irritability, and psychosis. Instances of dementia have been encountered.[188,201,222] "Mental dullness," often present since birth, is also observed in cases of pseudohypoparathyroidism.[69]

Wilson's Disease (Hepatolenticular Degeneration)

In 1912, Wilson described the clinical entity named after him.[257] Its clinical features are protean and are referable to the damage of the liver or central nervous system. They include evidence of liver failure, such as jaundice or ascites, and neurological symptoms or signs, such as rigidity, tremor, dystonic movements and postures, disturbances of speech and swallowing, and, infrequently, convulsions, transient coma, and "mental changes."[256] The latter may resemble, at times, schizophrenia[4,23] and in other instances may present as variable degrees of dementia, especially in the final stages.[49,50,89]

Wilson commented that the loss of intellectual functions may be more apparent than real, suggested by the "idiotic appearance" of the patients, to which may be added the interference with communication resulting from the dysarthria. He remarks that, "facility, docility, childishness, and emotional overaction form the chief features of the more chronic cases, together with a narrowing of the mental horizon."[256] In a psychological study[118] employing a battery of tests, seven patients with Wilson's disease all showed some "loss in the capacity for conceptual thinking," which was greatest in those patients with the longest duration of illness.

Wilson's disease is inherited as an autosomal recessive trait, and consanguinity is common in the ancestry of afflicted persons.[23]

Liver Disease

A permanent and progressive neurological disorder may be observed in persons suffering from chronic hepatic insufficiency.[246,250] The clinical features include—in addition to evidence of dementia—tremor, asterixis, ataxia, and speech disorder. Athetosis, chorea, and "action myoclonus" are encountered at times. The mental alteration is of variable degree and is characterized by defects in memory, abstracting ability, attentiveness, and concentration, accompanied by indolence and apathy.

The hepatic insufficiency may be due to cirrhosis, inflammatory disease, or surgical portacaval shunts. Victor, Adams, and Cole[246] found in all patients an elevation of the blood ammonia level or an abnormality on testing of the ammonium tolerance. While hepatic coma had occurred on one or more occasions in the majority of these patients, the relationship of the coma to the encephalopathy was variable. Coma preceded the evolution of the encephalopathy in some instances, while it occurred only after onset of the neurological disorder in other cases.

The significant neuropathological changes are a patchy necrosis at the junction of cerebral cortex and white matter and in the striatum, degeneration of neurons in cortex, cerebellum, and lentiform nuclei, and an increase in the size and number of protoplasmic astrocytes.

Hypoglycemia

Survivors of hypoglycemic attacks, regardless of cause (endogenous or exogenous insulin, functional hypoglycemia), may suffer permanent neurological damage, such as hemiplegia, aphasia, tremor and other extrapyramidal manifestations, and especially dementia and significant personality changes.[76,185] The pathological alterations in the brain resemble those produced by anoxia.

Remote Effects of Carcinoma

Dementia has been observed as part of the neurological syndrome associated with carcinoma.[30,136] In one series of 42 patients, progressive dementia accompanied other neurological disorders in 14 instances.[30] Mental alteration occurred with particular frequency in patients with cortical-cerebellar degeneration but was also encountered in some patients with peripheral neuropathy and other neuromuscular disorders. The progression of the dementia was variable.

In the majority of instances, pathological examination failed to show abnormalities capable of explaining the mental picture. Inflammatory changes were encountered in some cases, particularly in the subthalamic nuclei and in the nuclei of the brainstem.

The primary neoplasms were located in the lungs in the great majority of cases. The ovaries, prostate, rectum, and breasts were infrequently the site of the primary tumor.

Cushing's Syndrome

Psychiatric disturbances are common in Cushing's syndrome[207,235] and range from fatigability and irritability to psychotic degrees of derangement, in particular severe depressions. Mental dullness is observed at times, which may be coupled with some memory impairment. Substantial improvement may follow appropriate treatment, although progressive dementia following radiation therapy of the pituitary region has been reported.[207]

Uremia

Renal failure is frequently accompanied by neurological features, including myoclonus and fasciculations, tremor, asterixis, convulsions, muscular alterations, and evidence of peripheral neuropathy.[131,236] Emotional lability, irritability, and confusional states are common and may at times progress to impairment of memory, both for remote and recent events, failure to assimilate new material, disturbance of comprehension, abstraction, and orientation. Korsakoff's psychosis and Wernicke's encephalopathy may be encountered, particularly in instances with superimposed nutritional deficiency. In

179

cases amenable to therapy, reversal of the neurological and mental disturbances is the usual consequence.

VASCULAR DISORDERS

Arteriosclerosis

The diagnosis of "arteriosclerotic dementia" is frequently made in instances of gradual reduction of intellectual capacities, particularly if evidence of systemic or retinal arteriosclerosis is available. There is good evidence that this diagnosis is not justified by the facts in a large percentage of cases.

The degree of correlation between systemic, retinal, and cerebral arteriosclerosis has been reported to be of a low order.[11] Equally, the correlation of the degree of cerebrovascular arteriosclerosis and dementia is limited. In one study,[179] no difference was found in the character, location, and degree of arteriosclerotic changes between demented and nondemented elderly persons. The high incidence of senile plaques and neurofibrillary changes in elderly demented persons[64,180,232] suggests that many of these persons are suffering from a parenchymatous degenerative disorder, i.e., Alzheimer's disease.

Using a different approach combining psychiatric techniques and cerebral blood flow studies, Butler[35] also concluded that factors other than arteriosclerosis have to be advanced to explain the organic brain syndrome of many elderly persons.

Whether "little strokes," or strokes not recognizable as such by sudden clinical alterations, will produce dementia, is yet uncertain. Fisher,[64] in discussing lacunar infarcts, states, "There is no doubt that as the number of lacunes increases producing the lacunar state (or état lacunaire), mental deterioration does occur." He suggests, however, that this rarely develops in a gradual fashion similar to senile dementia, but that a careful history will usually disclose information of some sudden changes. He further underlines the experience that involuntary laughing and crying point to vascular disease and are not observed in Alzheimer's disease or senile dementia.

Dementia is observed in instances of unilateral or bilateral carotid artery disease.[39,52,65,66,171,172,199] The incidence of dementia in bilateral carotid artery occlusion has been reported to be 29 per cent in 69 patients reviewed from the world literature but has been higher in other studies.[52,199] Three possible mechanisms may be responsible for the production of the intellectual deficit:

1. The longstanding interference with cerebral blood flow, with resultant decompensation of neuronal function and eventual cell loss.

2. Recurrent embolization of cholesterol or platelet material with resultant microinfarctions.

3. Infarction of cerebral tissue, in particular in the border zones, i.e., areas of overlap in the distribution of major cerebral vessels.

It is doubtful whether at present a clear answer can be provided. Certainly, a number of cases are on record in which there was good retention of intellectual faculties in the presence of bilateral occlusive disease. The clinical picture depends undoubtedly on the adequacy of the collateral circulation.[62] Surgical treatment, i.e., endarterectomy, has had beneficial results in some cases.[52,171,254]

Inflammatory Disease of Blood Vessels

DISSEMINATED LUPUS ERYTHEMATOSUS. Both neurological and psychiatric dysfunction are common in disseminated lupus.[81] The neurological manifestations include convulsions, hemiplegia, aphasia, and disorders of cranial and peripheral nerves. In the psychiatric sphere, depression and schizophreniform psychoses are encountered, but the most common finding is an "organic mental syndrome," characterized by confusion, disorientation, memory deficits, and visual and auditory hallucinations.[162,214] The development of these mental changes is not related to the administration of steroids or the presence of uremia.

THROMBOANGIITIS OBLITERANS. Thromboangiitis obliterans or Buerger's disease is a disputed entity. It is said to involve cerebral vessels in up to 20 per cent of cases.[81] Clinically, episodes of transient focal dysfunction may gradually lead to diffuse reduction of intellectual function.

Aortic Arch Syndrome ("Pulseless Disease")

Aortic arch syndrome is a broad term designating obliteration of the arteries arising from the convexity of the aorta. The causes include arteriosclerosis, syphilitic aortitis, and an inflammatory arteritis, known also as *Takayasu's arteritis*. The neurological features are manifold[44, 217] and include pulse irregularities or pulselessness, convulsions, visual disturbances, focal cerebral infarctions, memory impairment, and dementia.[4, 241]

Binswanger's Disease ("Subcortical Arteriosclerotic Encephalopathy")

Binswanger's disease is the term assigned to the pathological finding of severe atrophy of the cerebral white matter, affecting one or many convolutions of the hemispheres. The clinical features of the eight cases forming the basis of Binswanger's presentation were progressive dementia, beginning between 50 and 65 years of age, coupled with signs of focal cerebral disease. These included hemiparesis, hemianesthesia, hemianopsia, or aphasia. The focal disturbances presented in an apoplectiform manner and included convulsive episodes. The progression of the disease was a slow one, extending usually over more than 10 years. Binswanger described only the macroscopic changes in his cases. Most of the small number of patients reported subsequently had arteriosclerosis with prominent involvement of the small arteries supplying the white matter and accompanied by areas of demyelination.[47, 164] The coexistence of arteriosclerosis and a demyelinating process has been considered coincidental by some, who view the process as related to other demyelinating diseases.[156] Because of this confusion, it has been suggested that, "obscure cases of subcortical demyelination which are not clearly related to arteriosclerotic changes should not be associated with the name of Binswanger," and that moreover the term *subcortical arteriosclerotic encephalopathy* should be adopted.[164]

Arteriovenous Malformations

Psychiatric alterations, in particular reduction of intellectual capacities, have been observed in 50 per cent or more of patients with arteriovenous malformations.[163, 233] The aberration is variable and extends from mild derangements to severe dementia. Progressive brain atrophy due to shunting of blood through the arteriovenous malformation is believed to be responsible for the mental alterations,[163] but destruction of brain tissue by hemorrhage and blocking of the CSF-pathways due to adhesive arachnoiditis following subarachnoid hemorrhage may well be contributing factors.[234]

HYPOXIA AND ANOXIA

Reduction of oxygen supply to the central nervous system leads to neuronal dysfunction and, eventually, to death of nerve cells. According to the mechanism responsible, different types of anoxia may be classified:[41, 210]

1. Anemic or ischemic anoxia occurs mainly after cardiac arrest and complete circulatory arrest, such as strangulation, and in severe anemia or hemorrhage.

2. Anoxic anoxia is the result of decreased oxygen tension in circulating blood. Its causes include reduction of respiratory capacity (central or neuropathic respiratory failure, occlusion of airways by mechanical factor or disease processes, asthma), reduction of oxygen tension in the inspired air (resulting from high altitude, anesthesia, or exposure to poisonous fumes), or impaired oxygen saturation of blood due to cardiovascular anomalies.

3. Stagnant anoxia results from reduced oxygen delivery to the brain because of slowing of the circulation, in such conditions as cardiac failure and polycythemia.

4. Histotoxic anoxia is the condition in which the cells cannot utilize the available oxygen because of interference by toxic substances (cyanide poisoning, chronic alcoholism,[41] or lack of substrate, such as hypoglycemia.[185])

The gray matter of the brain is more severely affected by oxygen lack than the white matter, and preferential destruction of nerve cells is observed in the globus pallidus, corpus Luysi, striatum, visual cortex, and Ammon's horn. The location and nature of neuronal destruction vary considerably and depend at least in some measure on the type of anoxia, its severity, and its duration. Complete oxygen deprivation in vulnerable areas of the brain for more than 4 to 5 minutes leads to cell death,[210] but even lesser periods of oxygen lack may lead to neuronal changes.[149] Recovery from an anoxic episode, regardless of cause, may be complete or partial. Residual neurological features include a variety of focal neurological signs, such as hemiparesis, athetosis, parkinsonism, aphasia, apraxia, and agnosia. Varying degrees of dementia are encountered.[41, 175, 185] Neurological deterioration is at times observed following a period of recovery and beginning 7 to 21 days after the acute anoxic episode or exposure to carbon monoxide.[176, 185] While this event has been most commonly observed after carbon monoxide poisoning, it has also been encountered after anesthesia, cardiac arrest, and hypoglycemia.

Pathologically, the brain in such patients shows diffuse hemispheric demyelination with sparing of the subcortical connecting fibers and most of the neuronal mantle, which remains remarkably unscathed. There is a high mortality in such delayed reactions, and the majority of the survivors suffer a moderate to severe dementia.[176]

NORMAL PRESSURE HYDROCEPHALUS

Progressive dementia, accompanying communicating hydrocephalus with a normal or near-normal pressure of the cerebrospinal fluid, has been recognized as a potentially treatable condition in recent years.[2, 68, 93, 102, 148] In addition to the slowly progressive dementia, gait disturbances — ataxic or apractic in nature — and incontinence have been observed in many of the reported cases. The condition may develop without recognizable preceding events or may follow subarachnoid hemorrhage, trauma, or chronic meningitis or may accompany neoplasms.

Pneumoencephalographic examination demonstrates dilatation of the ventricular system, without evidence of obstruction, but with little or no air over the convexity of the hemispheres. The diagnosis is confirmd by isotope-encephalography,[20, 130] which demonstrates isotope concentration in the ventricular system. In instances of ventricular dilatation secondary to cerebral atrophy the isotope is not concentrated in the ventricles in a similar manner.

Some patients with this condition may improve temporarily after lumbar puncture or pneumoencephalography, while abrupt worsening following these procedures has been encountered in other instances.

Shunt procedures (lumboperitoneal or ventriculoatrial) have benefited a significant proportion of the reported patients, the degree of improvement ranging from a resumption of self-care to a return to the premorbid occupation. Some measure of improvement has also been reported to follow shunt procedures in parenchymatous degenerative brain diseases.[13] The pathophysiology of the condition is yet unclear. As a hypothesis, it has been suggested that, in the presence of enlargement of the ventricular system, the total force exerted on the ventricular walls will be increased even in the face of "normal" spinal fluid pressure, since the force acting upon the ventricular wall is the product of pressure times surface area. If this "hydraulic press effect" exceeds the elasticity of the brain tissue, enlargement of the ventricles will ensue. The validity of this concept has been contested,[77] since it fails to take into consideration the structural properties of the ventricular walls.

DEFICIENCY DISEASES

Wernicke-Korsakoff Syndrome

Mental disturbance is almost ubiquitous in the Wernicke syndrome and was absent in only 10 per cent of the patients of a large series.[245] Several different types of mental abnormalities were observed.

1. Delirium tremens.

2. Korsakoff's psychosis.

3. A state of indifference and apathy, with limited attention span and inability to concentrate, disorientation in place and time, and impairment of memory and judgment. Treatment with thiamine may improve the patient's alertness and attentiveness, and the features of Korsakoff's psychosis may become more apparent.

The memory defect is the most prominent feature of Korsakoff's psychosis and expresses itself as an inability to incorporate new information into the store of knowledge. In addition, there is difficulty in proper sequential ordering of past events;[247] the patient can no longer differentiate temporal foreground and background, resulting in confabulation, the juxtaposition of temporally unrelated events. Beyond the impairment of memory formation, disturbances in cognitive functions and concept formation have been demonstrated in patients with Korsakoff's psychosis.[225,226] Treatment with thiamine results in variable degrees of recovery, ranging from complete restoration of intellectual functions to socially incapacitating degrees of mental impairment.

Pellagra

Nicotinic acid deficiency in its full-blown form produces the clinical triad of pellagra, including dermatitis, diarrhea, and mental changes. It is probable that the deficiency of other vitamins plays a role in the clinical manifestations of the disease. The mental abnormalities cover a wide range and include depression, apathy, irritability, confusional and delirious states, and dementia. Other neurological manifestations include spasticity, ataxia, hyperreflexia, visual disturbances and peripheral neuropathy.[208]

Marchiafava-Bignami Disease

Marchiafava-Bignami disease is a rare disorder characterized pathologically by necrosis of the central portions of the corpus callosum. The main impact of the process affects the rostral part of the corpus callosum, but degeneration of the anterior and posterior commissures, the centrum semiovale, and the middle cerebellar peduncles has also been observed.[147]

Since it was first reported in 1903, less than 100 cases have been accumulated in the literature. The majority have been in males of Italian stock, but persons of different ethnic background, and a few women, have also been afflicted.[109] Excessive alcoholic intake, particularly of red wine, has been recorded in most instances, and an etiological relationship to this beverage has been suspected. This supposition cannot be upheld, however, since the disease has been observed in persons consuming other types of alcoholic beverages, as well as persons without any history of alcoholic abuse.[109] The disease is probably directly or indirectly due to a nutritional imbalance or avitaminosis, but the exact pathogenesis is unclear.

The clinical manifestations may begin suddenly or insidiously, and may be precipitated by a bout of drinking or an infection. Bilateral stiff-legged gait disturbances may usher in the disease, or the patient may fall without recognizable reason. In other instances, mental alterations, such as delirium, stupor, agitation, or progressive dementia, may mark the onset of the disorder and may be followed by focal or generalized convulsions, aphasia, apraxia, muscular rigidity, tremors, or hemiparesis. The illness lasts from a few days to several months. The clinical picture is usually progressive and is not usually influenced by any therapeutic measures, although recovery with vitamin B therapy has been reported in one case.[128] The correct diagnosis is usually made only at the time of postmortem examination.

Vitamin B_{12} and Folate Deficiency

Mild mental changes are commonly observed in vitamin B_{12} deficiency[70,204] and may be present before any abnormalities can be observed in blood or bone marrow.[60,219] The mental alterations include confusion, depression, irritability, and forgetfulness, and paranoid features are stressed by some authors. Progressive failure of all intellectual functions is encountered at times. The psychiatric changes may develop independent from other neurological manifestations of the disease but are accompanied by EEG changes.[60] Significant improvement or complete restoration of function can be expected with vitamin B_{12} therapy. Improvement after folic acid therapy in two demented patients has led to the suggestion that folate deficiency may also cause intellectual deterioration.[218]

TOXINS AND DRUGS

A large number of drugs and exogenous toxins affect the central nervous system. Frequently, contact with these agents produces an "acute brain syndrome," characterized by disturbances of mentation, alterations of perception and behavior, and emotional instability. In some instances, a chronic illness may develop, usually characterized by impairment of orientation, memory, and general intellectual performance.

Metals

Lead intoxication, in the adult usually the result of industrial exposure, produces an encephalopathy characterized by irritability, memory impairment, disorientation, and drowsiness. Convulsions are commonly observed, and coma may supervene.[14,149,256]

Mental alterations occur also in mercury intoxication, particularly after exposure to organic mercury compounds.[121] The epidemic occurrence of a neurological disorder in Minamata Bay, Japan, is thought to be due to an organic mercury compound. Clinical symptoms and signs in afflicted persons include incoordination, involuntary movements, signs of corticospinal tract dysfunction, and variable degrees of emotional and intellectual disorders.[121]

Manganese poisoning, occurring mainly in miners, produces features of a disorder of the extrapyramidal system, with severe tremors, muscular rigidity, and a disturbance of gait.[1] Psychosis has been observed, as well as severe mental deterioration.[149]

Organic Compounds

The majority of organic compounds capable of affecting the nervous system produce an acute toxic picture, frequently resulting in death. Prolonged effects, with mental deterioration, follow exposure to nitrobenzenes, aniline compounds, bromine hydrocarbons, and tri-ortho-cresyl-phosphate,[17] and prolonged exposure to carbon disulfide[17] and carbon tetrachloride.[215]

Carbon Monoxide

Recovery from the acute stage of carbon monoxide poisoning may be followed, at times after a period of relative well-being lasting 7 to 21 days, by progressive deterioration of neurological functions, with dementia, Korsakoff's psychosis, manic or depressive states, and features resembling Parkinson's disease.[41,176,197] Gradual recovery, complete or partial, may take place. Mental dullness, depression, and memory deficits may also result from chronic exposure to small concentrations of carbon monoxide.[79,256]

Drugs

Reduction of mental functions, sufficient to suggest chronic brain disease, follows the prolonged and excessive use of bromides, paraldehyde, or barbiturates. Other signs suggesting drug intoxication, such as drowsiness, ataxia, slurring of speech, or hallucinations, may assist in the diagnosis but at times may be lacking. Marked reduction of psychomotor activity and retardation of thought processes may also accrue from the use of the tranquilizing drugs.

It has been suggested that the major anticonvulsive drugs, diphenylhydantoin (Dilantin), primidone (Mysoline), as well as phenobarbital, are capable of producing various neurological alterations, including dementia, by their interference with the metabolism of folic acid and vitamin B_{12}.[183]

BRAIN TUMORS

The great frequency of mental and emotional disorders in patients with cerebral neoplasms has been reflected in many studies.[22,34,92,98,100,117,153,155,194,205,251] A detailed review of the available material here is not intended. There is throughout the literature a continuing thread of argument concerning the specificity, or its lack, of the psychiatric derangement according to the tumor location, extent, or histological characteristics. The problem is compounded by several difficulties, not the least of which results from the lack of sharp semantic definitions. The term *dementia* may well at times be too inclusive, for instance in cases showing a specific memory deficit akin to the Korsakoff syndrome. In other instances, faulty responses on the part of the patient may be the result of apathy and a reduced level of alertness, rather than an expression of specific conceptual difficulties.

In addition, the extent of the neoplasm and its effect on adjacent and remote parts of the brain is usually hard to determine. Edema, compression of neighboring structures, interference with cerebral blood flow, and the effect of increased intracranial pressure on the entire central nervous system contribute to the emerging clinical picture. Moreover, the cerebral localization of intellectual functions is still poorly understood,[174] and the study of brain tumors is not particularly suitable to enlarge the available body of information concerning this point. Wilson[256] went so far as to say that, "Most analyses and allocations of mental syndromes accompanying cerebral tumors are worthless."

Mental or behavioral alterations in general occur in 50 to 70 per cent of all brain tumors.[194,205,249,251] Dementia, or memory loss, has been reported in instances of neoplasms involving, in particular, the frontal lobes,[10,71,155] but also in tumors of the third ventricle and hypothalamus,[187,209,255] thalamus,[5,224] the occipital lobes,[7,72,194] parietal lobes,[194] temporal lobes,[119] and corpus callosum.[9,18,154] Many of these reports seek to relate a specific mental disorder with the involved area.

An opposing view is held by Walther-Büel,[251] who based his conclusions on 600 cases of brain tumors, 60 of which he examined personally. He found it possible to divide the mental disorders encountered into two broad categories.

1. "Chronic organic psychosyndromes," with prominent memory disturbance, little or no disturbance of attentiveness, affective lability, and a high degree of fatigability in all mental performances.

2. Disturbances of consciousness with prominent reduction of attentiveness, inability to concentrate, and incoherence of thought, eventually progressing to torpor and stupor.

Both symptom constellations were encountered with equal frequency in the patient population studied and did not appear to be related to the location of the tumors in the brain. The organic psychosyndrome was infrequently encountered in children and young adults, but its incidence, as well as its severity, increased in the higher age groups. Disturbances of consciousness, on the other hand, were observed in all age groups, regardless of the location of the neoplasm.

Although specific changes in mentation cannot be correlated with brain tumors in various locations, dementia of recent onset must always alert the physician to the possibility of primary or secondary cerebral neoplasia and prompt complete evaluation to diagnose or exclude brain tumor.

TRAUMA

Open and Closed Head Injuries

Severe reduction of intellectual function is not a common result of head injuries.[38,91] Miller and Stern[152] reexamined 92 survivors of severe head injuries from 3 to 40 years after the initial insult. Some degree of dementia was present in 10 patients, but these authors concluded that, "major cerebral trauma is clearly statistically insignificant as a cause of dementia severe enough to demand long-term hospital care." In a Finnish study[103] of 3552 war-injured persons, followed for 22 to 26 years, Korsakoff's syndrome was observed in 23 survivors, and grave dementia in 11. In a Japanese study,[165] disorders of intellectual function were observed in 22 instances of 1168 cases of closed head injuries. Even after prolonged post-traumatic unconsciousness (in excess of 3 weeks), a socially disabling reduction of intellectual function is not the common end result, although some degree of intellectual deficit was observed in the majority of survivors.[242]

Disruption of nerve fibers by shearing forces has been postulated as a mechanism producing dementia in survivors of head injuries.[220]

Progressive dementia, as an expression of Alzheimer's disease, Pick's disease, or Creutzfeldt-Jakob disease, following head injury has been recorded.[40,220]

The Punch-Drunk Syndrome

An insidiously progressive cerebral disorder may develop in former boxers years after their ring career has ended.[43,144,206] The number of fights, in particular the number of head blows and knockouts, appears to bear a relation to the syndrome, which is characterized by dementia ("dementia pugilistica"), cerebellar and extrapyramidal dysfunction. Convulsions occur in some affected persons. Pneumoencephalographic studies show cerebral atrophy, and abnormalities of the septum pellucidum have been seen in a high percentage of cases.[144] The neuropathological alterations are those of multiple cortical infarcts or of Alzheimer's disease.[220]

Subdural Hematoma

The gradual accumulation of blood in the subdural space may be accompanied by a reduction of intellectual functions, similar to that observed in patients with brain tumors. In particular in the elderly, the clinical course of subdural hematoma may resemble parenchymatous degenerative disease.[173,221] A demented state may also be the end result in operated cases of subdural hematoma.[46] In elderly patients with a recent onset of progressive dementia, subdural hematoma should always be considered as a potential cause.

Heat Stroke

The acute hyperpyrexia of heat stroke may lead to severe neurological damage. Dementia is said to result in about 10 per cent of survivors of heat stroke.[256]

INFECTIONS

Brain Abscess

The psychiatric features of brain abscess may resemble those of brain tumors. Reduction of intellectual abilities may persist after surgical treatment.[227]

Bacterial Meningitis

Only rarely does acute bacterial meningitis in the adult leave significant residual intellectual impairment.[59,147,191] In one report concerning 99 patients with bacterial meningitis, permanent mental defects were seen in only 3 cases, all children.[51]

More severe neurological sequelae have been found after tuberculous meningitis, affecting 23 of 100 children surviving this disease.[132] Six of these children were profoundly mentally retarded, all showing other major neurological deficits as well. In adults, 11 of 178 patients surviving tuberculous meningitis for at least 1 year after start of treatment had "marked impairment of intellect, judgment, and skills."[58]

Fungal Meningitis

Acute or subacute mental disorders are common among the early signs of fungal meningitis, and in one study occurred in 3 of 7 patients with histoplasma meningitis, and in 26 patients with cryptococcal meningitis.[240] The mental features observed probably did not suggest dementia in the cases of histoplasma meningitis,[237] but confusion, personality changes, and memory defects were present in a small percentage of the cases of cryptococcal meningitis.[36]

Encephalitis

In most of the forms of viral encephalitis occurring in the Western world, serious effects on mental function in adults are usually transient, while persistent neurological and intellectual deficits may occur in children.[16,147] These sequelae are seen with greater frequency, and are more severe, in the Eastern equine form than in the St. Louis type or Western equine encephalitis.

Mental deterioration was found in 4 of 56 former U.S. servicemen who had survived an attack of Japanese B encephalitis.[90]

189

In contrast, severe mental disorders are frequently the end result in survivors of herpes simplex encephalitis and other forms of inclusion body encephalitis.[82,147] A progressive dementia has been observed in patients suffering from a subacute form of encephalitis affecting the limbic area.[31] Inclusion bodies were not seen in the histological material from these cases and only rarely in cases of chronic encephalitis with focal seizures and intellectual deterioration.[3]

In subacute sclerosing panencephalitis (SSPE), memory defects, along with behavioral changes, may be the initial sign of the developing disease.

Progressive Multifocal Leukoencephalopathy

A demyelinating disorder accompanying Hodgkin's disease and chronic lymphocytic leukemia was first recognized in 1958.[15] The term *progressive multifocal leukoencephalopathy* was used to describe the disorder. By 1964, Richardson[184] was able to review 45 cases, and others have been added to the literature since.

The disorder has been found not only in association with leukemia and lymphomas, but also with polycythemia vera, sarcoidosis, tuberculosis, Whipple's disease, and carcinomatosis. It is progressive and leads to death in a few weeks to months. The clinical features include evidence of disseminated nervous system lesions, manifested by variable neurological signs, such as ataxia, dysarthria, limb paresis, visual field defects or blindness, confusional states, progressive dementia, and coma. The cerebrospinal fluid is usually normal, while the EEG commonly shows nonspecific abnormalities.

The pathological changes consist of multiple areas of demyelination, with relative sparing of the axis cylinders. On theoretical grounds, the possibility was advanced that the disorder may be due to viral action in individuals with impaired immune responses.[184] The presence of virus-like particles in glial cells of patients with this disease was first reported in 1964[260] and has since been confirmed in other cases.

Behçet's Syndrome

Behçet's syndrome is a rare entity, possibly of viral origin. Its main clinical characteristics include ulcerations of the mouth and genitalia, and iritis. Other frequent manifestations are erythema nodosum, thrombophlebitis, a nonspecific skin sensitivity, and neurological involvement, which occurs in about 25 per cent of cases. The illness affects preferentially young males and tends to run a protracted, remitting course, although slow progression may also be observed.

The neurological features include headaches, pleocytosis, signs of involvement of the brainstem, spasticity, and parkinsonism.[248] Intellectual deterioration is encountered at times. Claims for a viral etiology of this disorder are yet unconfirmed.[147,248]

Kuru

A peculiar neurological disease among the Fore tribesmen of New Guinea was first recognized in 1957 by Gajdusek and Zigas.[74] The disease, which affects primarily adult females and children of both sexes, begins with disturbances of locomotion and shaking of the head and extremities. In the further evolution of the disorder, chorea or athetosis, lability of emotional expression, disturbances of extraocular movements and progressive signs of cerebellar involvement appear. The total duration of the illness is less than 2 years, and dementia develops frequently in the late stages.[107]

Gajdusek, Gibbs, and Alpers[73] were able to produce experimentally a disease resembling kuru clinically and pathologically in chimpanzees inoculated with brain tissue derived from kuru patients, and to repeat the process by second and third passages. There is strong evidence that kuru may be the clinical result of infection with a slow-growing virus, possibly transmitted by the tribal custom of cannibalism.[114]

Lues

Dementia paralytica, or general paresis, is due to direct invasion of the brain by Treponema pallidum, which leads to cortical atrophy, with thickening of the leptomeninges. Once one of the leading causes for admission to mental institutions, fresh instances of the disease are now infrequently encountered.

Men are affected more frequently than women, and the disease usually declares itself 10 to 20 years after the initial luetic infection. In the period before modern treatment of syphilitic infections, it was estimated that approximately 5 per cent of persons with untreated syphilis would develop dementia paralytica.[147,256]

The onset is usually a gradual one, although it may be marked in a more dramatic manner by convulsions or a stroke-like event. Minor alterations in conduct, errors in judgment, carelessness in personal appearance, instability, mood swings, depressive or hypomanic features mark the initial deviation from the previous state of health. The disease process may travel along several different roads, and a number of clinical subtypes have been enumerated.[256] The common denominator, however, is the attrition of intellectual, social, and moral capacities. Other features such as euphoria, megalomania, depression, agitation, and apathy are only variations on the basic theme. Signs of neurological disease, such as tremors, dysarthria, pupillary changes, or ataxia, may accompany the personality disintegration but may be absent or provide only a dim background to the central events. The serological tests for syphilis in blood and spinal fluid are nearly always positive and serve to set this disease apart from other dementing processes. Treatment of general paresis with penicillin cures the disease and often has some beneficial effect on the dementia.

191

OTHER DISEASES

Multiple Sclerosis

Significant intellectual deterioration is uncommon in the early stages of multiple sclerosis, but features of organic brain disease emerge frequently as the disease progresses.[19,190] On psychological tests, the loss of abstracting ability has been found to approximate the extent of neurological damage.[168] In the majority of instances, alterations in the affective sphere are more prominent than intellectual deterioration. Rarely a marked progressive dementia has been recorded.[24,256]

Muscular Dystrophy

Among patients with progressive muscular dystrophy, mental deficiency is encountered with greater frequency than in other disabling disorders.[8,160,189,259] It is probable that this mental defect is a nonprogressive one, in contrast to that encountered in myotonic muscular dystrophy. Intellectual deterioration and social descent are observed in this disorder with considerable frequency.[135] Thomasen[231] found in many of his myotonic cases mental defects dating back to early childhood. Moreover, he observed progressive intellectual deterioration in one third of his patients, particularly those in whom the clinical manifestations of the disease became first apparent in childhood. The cause of this deterioration is not yet understood, but pneumoencephalographic evidence of ventricular enlargement has been presented.[182]

Whipple's Disease

Whipple's disease is an uncommon disorder, characterized clinically by weakness, weight loss, steatorrhea, and polyarthritis, and pathologically by the accumulation of PAS-positive material in the macrophages of the intestinal mucosa and in the mesenteric lymph nodes.

The disease affects mainly middle-aged males. Neurological manifestations have been reported, including dysarthria, ophthalmoplegia, ataxia, myoclonus, and dementia.[123,216] The neuropathological findings were those of a nodular encephalitis, with accumulation of PAS-positive material.[216] Progressive multifocal leukoencephalopathy has also been reported in association with Whipple's disease.[184]

Concentration-Camp Syndrome

In a number of survivors of severe nutritional deprivation in European concentration camps, progressive mental changes were observed. These presented originally as neurotic manifestations, with signs of organic brain disease later supervening. The pneumoencephalogram showed evidence of cerebral atrophy.[55,253]

GENETIC ASPECTS OF DEMENTIA

Several of the diseases producing dementia appear—at least in some cases—to be determined by genetic factors. The evidence for genetic transmission is strong in some diseases but is much more tentative in relatively rare conditions. Still in other diseases, the principle of "genetic heterogeneity" appears to operate, which states that phenotypic similarity may be produced by genotypically different conditions.

For detailed evaluation of the available evidence, reference is made to the monograph *The Genetics of Neurological Disorders,* by R. T. C. Pratt.[178] There can be little doubt that further epidemiological studies will modify the present state of knowledge as summarized in Table 2.

Table 2. Genetic aspects of dementia

Disease	Mode of Transmission	References	Remarks
Alzheimer's	Dominant or multifactorial	61, 101, 178, 203	Genetic factors apparent in only a limited number of instances.
Pick's	Dominant-autosomal	178, 203, 243	Genetic factors apparent in only a limited number of instances.
Creutzfeldt-Jakob	Dominant-autosomal	146	Only three familial instances.
Huntington's chorea	Dominant-autosomal	178	
Senile dementia	Dominant or multifactorial	178	Risk of relative of propositi is four times the risk of general population.
Hallervorden-Spatz	Undetermined		Only few instances of familial occurrence recorded.
Spino-cerebellar degenerations	Variable	6, 37, 88, 140, 169, 178, 202	
Myoclonus-epilepsy (Lafora-type)	Autosomal recessive	95, 96	
Wilson's	Autosomal recessive	178, 257	

REFERENCES

1. ABD EL NABY, S., AND HASSANEIN, M.: *Neuropsychiatric manifestations of chronic manganese poisoning.* J. Neurol. Neurosurg. Psychiat. 28:282, 1965.

2. ADAMS, R. D., FISHER, C. M., HAKIM, S., OJEMANN, R. G., AND SWEET, W. H.: *Symptomatic occult hydrocephalus with "normal" cerebrospinal fluid pressure.* New Eng. J. Med. 273:117, 1965.

3. AGUILAR, M. J., AND RASMUSSEN, T.: *Role of encephalitis in pathogenesis of epilepsy.* Arch. Neurol. 2:663, 1960.

4. AITA, J. A.: *Neurologic Manifestations of General Diseases.* Charles C Thomas, Publisher, Springfield, Ill., 1964.

5. AJURIAGUERRA, J. DE, HÉCAEN, H., AND SADOUN, R.: *Les troubles mentaux au cours des tumeurs de la région méso-diencéphalique.* L'Encéphale 43:406, 1954.

6. AKELAITIS, A. J.: *Hereditary form of primary parenchymatous atrophy of cerebellar cortex associated with mental deterioration.* Amer. J. Psychiat. 94:1115, 1938.

7. ALLEN, I. M.: *A clinical study of tumours involving the occipital lobe.* Brain 53:194, 1930.

8. ALLEN, T. D., AND RODGIN, D. W.: *Mental retardation in association with progressive muscular dystrophy.* Amer. J. Dis. Child. 100:208, 1960.

9. ALPERS, B. J.: *A note on the mental syndrome of corpus callosum tumors.* J. Nerv. Ment. Dis. 84:621, 1936.

10. ALPERS, B. J.: *Clinical Neurology,* ed. 5. F. A. Davis Co., Philadelphia, 1963.

11. ALPERS, B. J., FORSTER, F. M., AND HERBERT, P. A.: *Retinal, cerebral and systemic arteriosclerosis. A histopathologic study.* Arch. Neurol. Psychiat. 60:440, 1948.

12. ALZHEIMER, A.: *Über eine eigenartige Erkrankung der Hirnrinde.* Centralblatt Nervenheilk. Psychiat. 18:177, 1907.

13. APPENZELLER, O., AND SALMON, J. H.: *Treatment of parenchymatous degeneration of the brain by ventriculo-atrial shunting of the cerebrospinal fluid.* J. Neurosurg. 26:478, 1967.

14. ARING, C. D., AND TRUFANT, S. A.: Effects of heavy metals on the central nervous system. Proc. Assn. Res. Nerv. Ment. Dis. 32:463, 1953.

15. ASTRÖM, K. E., MANCALL, E. L., AND RICHARDSON, E. P., JR.: *Progressive multifocal leukoencephalopathy; a hitherto unrecognized complication of chronic lymphocytic leukaemia and Hodgkin's disease.* Brain 81:93, 1958.

16. BAKER, A. B.: Viral encephalitis, Chap. 17 in Baker, A. B. (ed.): *Clinical Neurology,* ed 2. Hoeber-Harper, New York, 1962.

17. BAKER, A. B., AND TICHY, F. Y.: The effects of the organic solvents and industrial poisonings on the central nervous system. Proc. Assn. Res. Nerv. Ment. Dis. 32:475, 1953.

18. BALDUZZI, O.: *Die Tumoren des Corpus callosum.* Arch. Psychiat. Nervenheilk. 79:1, 1927.

19. BALDWIN, M. V.: *A clinico-experimental investigation into the psychologic aspects of multiple sclerosis.* J. Nerv. Ment. Dis. 115:299, 1952.

20. BANNISTER, R., GILFORD, E., AND KOCEN, R.: *Isotope encephalography in the diagnosis of dementia due to communicating hydrocephalus.* Lancet 2:1014, 1967.

21. BARTTER, F. C.: *The parathyroid gland and its relationship to diseases of the nervous system.* Proc. Assn. Res. Nerv. Ment. Dis. 32:1, 1953.

22. BARUK, H.: *Les troubles mentaux dans les tumeurs cérébrales.* Thèse, G. Doin et Cie, édit., Paris, 1926.

23. BEARN, A. G.: Wilson's Disease, in Stanbury, J. B., Wyngaarden, J. B., and Fredrickson, D. S. (eds.) : *The Metabolic Basis of Inherited Disease,* ed. 2. McGraw-Hill Book Co., New York, 1966.

24. BERGIN, J. D.: *Rapidly progressing dementia in disseminated sclerosis.* J. Neurol. Neurosurg. Psychiat. 20:285, 1957.

25. BERLIN, L.: *Presenile sclerosis (Alzheimer's disease) with features resembling Pick's disease.* Arch. Neurol. Psychiat. 61:369, 1949.

26. BITTENBENDER, J. B., AND QUADFASEL, F. A.: *Rigid and akinetic forms of Huntington's chorea.* Arch. Neurol. 7:275, 1962.

27. BLESSED, G., TOMLINSON, B. E., AND ROTH, M.: *The association between quantitative measures of dementia and of senile change in the cerebral grey matter of elderly subjects.* Brit. J. Psychiat. 114:797, 1968.

28. BLINDERMAN, E. E., WEIDNER, W., AND MARKHAM, C. H.: *The pneumoencephalogram in Huntington's chorea.* Neurology 14:601, 1964.

29. BLUMENTHAL, H., AND MILLER, C.: *Motor nuclear involvement in progressive supranuclear palsy.* Arch. Neurol. 20:362, 1969.

30. BRAIN, R., AND HENSON, R. A.: *Neurological syndromes associated with carcinoma.* Lancet 2:971, 1958.

31. BRIERLEY, J. B., CORSELLIS, J. A. N., HIERONS, R., AND NEVIN, S.: *Subacute encephalitis of later adult life. Mainly affecting the limbic areas.* Brain 83:357, 1960.

32. BROWNELL, B., AND OPPENHEIMER, D. R.: *An ataxic form of subacute presenile polioencephalopathy (Creutzfeldt-Jakob disease).* J. Neurol. Neurosurg. Psychiat. 28:350, 1965.

33. BRUYN, G. W., MINK, C. J. K., AND CALJÉ, J. F.: *Biochemical studies in Huntington's chorea.* Neurology 15:455, 1965.

34. BUSCH, E.: *Psychical symptoms in neurosurgical disease.* Acta Psychiat. Neurol. Scand. 15:257, 1940.

35. BUTLER, R. N.: Psychiatric aspects of cerebrovascular disease in the aged. Proc. Assn. Res. Nerv. Ment. Dis. 41:255, 1961.

36. BUTLER, W. T., ALLING, D. W., SPICKARD, A., AND UTZ, J. P.: *Diagnostic and prognostic value of clinical and laboratory findings in cryptococcal meningitis.* New Eng. J. Med. 270:59, 1964.

37. CARTER, H. G., AND SUKAVAJANA, C.: *Familial cerebello-olivary degeneration with late development of rigidity and dementia.* Neurology 6:876, 1956.

38. CAVENESS, W. F.: Posttraumatic sequelae, in Caveness, W. R., and Walker, A. E. (eds.) : *Head Injury Conference Proceedings.* J. B. Lippincott Co., Philadelphia, 1966, Chap. 17.

39. CLARKE, E., AND HARRISON, C. V.: *Bilateral carotid artery obstruction.* Neurology 6:705, 1956.

40. CORSELLIS, J. A. N., AND BRIERLEY, J. B.: *Observations on the pathology of insidious dementia following head injury.* J. Ment. Sci. 105:714, 1959.

41. COURVILLE, C. B.: Cerebral anoxia, in Baker, A. B. (ed.) : *Clinical Neurology*. Hoeber-Harper, New York, 1962, Chap. 12.

42. CREUTZFELDT, H. G.: *Über eine eigenartige herdförmige Erkrankung des Zentralnervensystems*. Z. ges. Neurol. Psychiat. 57:1, 1920.

43. CRITCHLEY, M.: *Medical aspects of boxing, particularly from a neurological viewpoint*. Brit. Med. J. 1:357, 1957.

44. CURRIER, R. D., DEJONG, R. N., AND BOLE, G. G.: *Pulseless disease: Central nervous system manifestations*. Neurology 4:818, 1954.

45. DAVID, N. J., MACKEY, E. A., AND SMITH, J. L.: *Further observations in progressive supranuclear palsy*. Neurology 18:349, 1968.

46. DAVIES, F. L.: *Mental abnormalities following subdural hematoma*. Lancet 1:1369, 1960.

47. DAVISON, C.: *Progressive subcortical encephalopathy. (Binswanger's disease)*. J. Neuropath. Exp. Neurol. 1:42, 1948.

48. DEMYER, W., HARTER, D. H., AND ZEMAN, W.: *Familial spasticity, hyperkinesia and dementia*. Acta Neuropath. 4:28, 1964.

49. DENNY-BROWN, D.: *Abnormal copper metabolism and hepatolenticular degeneration*. Proc. Assn. Res. Nerv. Ment. Dis. 32:190, 1952.

50 DENNY-BROWN, D., AND PORTER, H.: *The effect of BAL (2, 3-dimercaptopropanol) on hepatolenticular degeneration (Wilson's disease)*. New Eng. J. Med. 245:917, 1951.

51. DODGE, P. R., AND SWARTZ, M. N.: *Bacterial meningitis—a review of selected aspects. II. Special neurologic problems, postmeningitis complications and clinicopathological correlations*. New Eng. J. Med. 272:1003, 1965.

52. DRAKE, W. E., JR., BAKER, M., BLUMENKRANTZ, J., AND DAHLGREN, H.: *The quality and duration of survival in bilateral carotid occlusive disease. A preliminary survey of the effect of thromboendarterectomy*. Transactions Sixth Conference on Cerebral Vascular Diseases. Grune & Stratton, Inc., New York, 1968.

53. EHRENTHEIL, O.: *Differential diagnosis of organic dementias and affective disorders in aged persons*. Geriatrics 12:426, 1957.

54. EIDEN, H. F., AND LECHNER, H.: *Über psychotische Zustandsbilder bei der Pickschen und Alzheimerschen Krankheit*. Arch. Psychiatr. Nervenkr. 184:393, 1950. Quoted from Sjögren et al. See Reference 203.

55. EITINGER, L.: *Concentration Camp Survivors in Norway and Israel*. Universitetsforlaget, Oslo, and Allen and Unwin, London, 1964.

56. ELIZAN, T. S., CHEN, K., MATHAI, K. V., DUNN, D., AND KURLAND, L. T.: *Amyotrophic lateral sclerosis and Parkinsonism-dementia complex*. Arch. Neurol. 14:347, 1966.

57. ELIZAN, T. S., HIRANO, A., ABRAMS, B. M., NEED, R. L., VANKUIS, C., AND KURLAND, L. T.: *Amyotrophic lateral sclerosis and Parkinsonism-dementia complex of Guam*. Arch. Neurol. 14:356, 1966.

58. FALK, A.: *Tuberculous meningitis in adults, with special reference to survival, neurologic residuals and work status*. Amer. Rev. Resp. Dis. 91:823, 1965.

59. FARMER, T. W.: *Neurologic complications during meningococcic meningitis treated with sulfonamide drugs.* Arch. Int. Med. 76:201, 1945.

60. FARMER, T. W.: Neurologic complications of vitamin and mineral disorders, in Baker, A. B. (ed.) : *Clinical Neurology.* Hoeber-Harper, New York, 1962, Chap. 44.

61. FELDMAN, R. G., CHANDLER, K. A., LEVY, L. L., AND GLASER, G. H.: *Familial Alzheimer's disease.* Neurology 13:811, 1963.

62. FIELDS, W. S., EDWARDS, W. H., AND CRAWFORD, E. S.: *Bilateral carotid artery thrombosis.* Arch. Neurol. 4:369, 1961.

63 FISHER, C. M.: *The clinical picture in Creutzfeldt-Jakob disease.* Trans. Amer. Neurol. Assn. 85:147, 1960.

64. FISHER, C. M.: *Dementia in cerebral vascular diseases.* Transactions Sixth Conference on Cerebral Vascular Diseases, Grune & Stratton, Inc., New York, 1968.

66. FISHER, M.: *Senile-dementia—a new explanation of its causation.* Canad. Med. Assn. J. 65:1, 1951.

65. FISHER, M.: *Occlusion of the carotid arteries.* Arch. Neurol. Psychiat. 72:187, 1954.

67. FOLEY, J. M., AND DENNY-BROWN, D.: *Subacute progressive bulbar myoclonus.* J. Neuropath. Exp. Neurol. 16:133, 1957.

68. FOLTZ, E. L., AND WARD, A. A.: *Communicating hydrocephalus from subarachnoid hemorrhage.* J. Neurosurg. 13:546, 1956.

69. FRAME, B., AND CARTER, S.: *Pseudohypoparathyroidism.* Neurology 5: 297, 1955.

70. FRASER, T. N.: *Cerebral manifestations of Addisonian pernicious anemia.* Lancet 2:458, 1960.

71. FRAZIER, C. H.: *Tumor involving the frontal lobe alone.* Arch. Neurol. Psychiat. 35:525, 1936.

72. FRAZIER, C. H., AND WAGGONER, R. W.: *Tumors of the occipital lobe.* Arch. Neurol. Psychiat. 22:1086, 1929.

73. GAJDUSEK, D. C., GIBBS, C. J., JR., AND ALPERS, M.: *Transmission and passage of experimental "kuru" to chimpanzees.* Science 155:212, 1967.

74. GAJDUSEK, D. C., AND ZIGAS, V.: *Kuru: Clinical, pathological and epidemiological study of an acute progressive degenerative disease of the central nervous system among natives of the Eastern Highland of New Guinea.* Amer. J. Med. 26:442, 1959.

75. GARCIN, R., BRION, S., AND KHOCHNEVIS, A.: *Le syndrome de Creutzfeldt-Jakob et les syndromes cortico-striés du presenium.* Rev. Neurol. 106: 506, 1962.

76. GAUTIER-SMITH, P. C.: Clinical aspects of hypoglycaemia, in Cumings, J. N., and Kremer, M. (eds.) : *Biochemical Aspects of Neurological Disorders,* 2nd ser. F. A. Davis Co. (Blackwell Scientific Publications), Philadelphia, 1965.

77. GESCHWIND, N.: *The mechanism of normal pressure hydrocephalus.* J. Neurol. Sci. 7:481, 1968.

78. GIBBS, C. J., GAJDUSEK, D. C., ASHER, D. M., ALPERS, M. P., BECK, E., DANIEL, P. M., AND MATTHEWS, W. B.: *Creutzfeldt-Jakob disease (spongiform encephalopathy): Transmission to the chimpanzee.* Science 161:388, 1968.

79. GILBERT, G. J., AND GLASER, G. H.: *Neurologic manifestations of chronic carbon monoxide poisoning.* New Eng. J. Med. 261:1217, 1959.

80. GILMAN, S., AND HORENSTEIN, S.: *Familial amyotrophic dystonic paraplegia.* Brain 87:51, 1964.

81. GLASER, G. H.: Neurologic complications of internal disease, in Baker, A. B., (ed.) : *Clinical Neurology,* Hoeber-Harper, New York 1962, Chap 46.

82. GLASER, G. H., SOLITAIRE, G. B., AND MANUELIDIS, E. E.: *Acute and subacute inclusion encephalitis.* Res. Publ. Assn. Res. Nerv. Ment. Dis. 44: 178, 1964.

83. GONATAS, N. K., TERRY, R. D., AND WEISS, M.: *Ultrastructural studies in Jakob-Creutzfeldt disease.* Trans. Amer. Neurol. Assn. 89:13, 1964.

84. GOODMAN, L.: *Alzheimer's disease.* J. Nerv. Ment. Dis. 117:97, 1953.

85. GOODMAN, R. M., HALL, C. L, JR., TERANGO, L., PERRINE, G. A., JR., AND ROBERTS, P. L.: *Huntington's chorea.* Arch. Neurol. 15:345, 1966.

86. GORDON, E. B., AND SIM, M.:*The EEG in presenile dementia.* J. Neurol. Neurosurg. Psychiat. 30:285, 1967.

87. GREEN, M. A., STEVENSON, L. D., FONSECA, J. E., AND WORTIS, S. B.: *Cerebral biopsy in patients with presenile dementia.* Dis. Nerv. Syst. 13: 303, 1952.

88. GREENFIELD, J. G.: *The Spino-Cerebellar Degenerations.* Charles C Thomas, Publisher, Springfield, Ill., 1954.

89. GREENFIELD, J. G.: in Blackwood, W., et al. (ed.) : *Greenfield's Neuropathology,* ed. 2. The Williams & Wilkins Co., Baltimore, 1966.

90. GROSSBERG, S., HEYMAN, A., AND KEEHN, R. J.: *Neurologic sequelae of Japanese encephalitis.* Trans. Amer. Neurol. Assn. 87:114, 1962.

91. GURDJIAN, E. S., AND WEBSTER, J. E.: *Head Injuries.* Little, Brown and Company, Boston, 1958.

92. GUVENER, A., BAGCHI, B. K., KOOI, K. A., AND CALHOUN, H. D.: *Mental and seizure manifestations in relation to brain tumors.* Epilepsia 5:166, 1964.

93. HAKIM, S., AND ADAMS, R. D.: *The special clinical problem of symptomatic hydrocephalus with normal cerebrospinal fluid pressure. Observations on cerebrospinal fluid hydrodynamics.* J. Neurol. Sci. 2:307, 1965.

94. HALLERVORDEN, J., AND SPATZ, H.: *Eigenartige Erkrankung im extrapyramidalen System mit besonderer Beteiligung des Globus pallidus und der Substantia nigra.* Z. ges. Neurol. Psychiat. 79:254, 1922.

95. HALLIDAY, A. M.: The clinical incidence of myoclonus, in Williams, D. (ed.): *Modern Trends in Neurology,* ed. 4. Appleton-Century-Crofts, New York, 1967.

96. HARRIMAN, D. G. F., AND MILLAR, J. H. D.: *Progressive familial myo-clonic epilepsy in three families: Its clinical features and pathological basis.* Brain 78:325, 1955.

97. HASLAM, M. T.: *Cellular magnesium levels and the use of penicillamine in the treatment of Huntington's chorea.* J. Neurol. Neurosurg. Psychiat. 30:185, 1967.

98. HÉCAEN, H. AND AJURIAGUERRA, J. DE: *Troubles mentaux au cours des tumeurs intracraniennes.* Masson et Cie, Paris, 1956.

99. HEIDENHAIN, A.: *Klinische und anatomische Untersuchungen über eine eigenartige organische Erkrankung des Zentralnervensystems im Praesenium.* Z. ges. Neurol. Psychiat. 118:49, 1928.

100. HENRY, G. W.: *Mental phenomena observed in cases of brain tumor.* Amer. J. Psychiat. 12:415, 1932.

101. HESTON, L. L., LOWTHER, D. L. W., AND LEVENTHAL, C. M.: *Alzheimer's disease.* Arch. Neurol. 15:225, 1966.

102. HILL, M. E., HOUGHEED, W. M., AND BARNETT, H. J. M.: *A treatable form of dementia due to normal-pressure, communicating hydrocephalus.* Canad. Med. Assn. J. 97:1309, 1967.

103. HILLBOM, E., AND CARHO, L.: Posttraumatic Korsakoff syndrome, in Walker, A. E., Caveness, W. F., and Critchley, M. (eds.): *The Late Effects of Head Injury.* Charles C Thomas, Publisher, Springfield, Ill., 1969.

104. HIRANO, A., KURLAND, L. T., KROOTH, R. S., AND LESSELL, S.: *Parkinsonism-dementia complex, an endemic disease on the island of Guam: I. Clinical features.* Brain 84:642, 1961.

105. HIRANO, A., MALAMUD, N., ELIZAN, T. S., AND KURLAND, L. T.: *Amyotrophic lateral sclerosis and Parkinsonism-dementia complex on Guam.* Arch. Neurol. 15:35, 1966.

106. HIRANO, A., MALAMUD, N., AND KURLAND, L. T.: *Parkinsonism-dementia complex, an endemic disease on the island of Guam: II. Pathological features.* Brain 84:662, 1961.

107. HORNABROOK, R. W.: *Kuru—a subacute cerebellar degeneration. The natural history and clinical features.* Brain 91:53, 1968.

108. HUNTINGTON, G.: *On chorea.* Med. and Surg. Reporter, Phila. 26:317, 1872.

109. IRONSIDE, R., BOSANQUET, F. D., AND MCMENEMEY, W. H.: *Central demyelination of the corpus callosum (Marchiafava-Bignami disease).* Brain 84:212, 1961.

110. JAKOB, A.: *Die extrapyramidalen Erkrankungen.* Springer, Berlin, 1923.

111. JANEWAY, R., RAVENS, J. R., PEARCE, L. A., ODOR, D. L., AND SUZUKI, K.: *Progressive myoclonus epilepsy with Lafora inclusion bodies. I. Clinical, genetic, histopathologic and biochemical aspects.* Arch. Neurol. 16:565, 1967.

112. JELLINEK, E. H.: *Fits, faints, coma and dementia in myxedema.* Lancet 2:1010, 1962.

113. JERVIS, G. A.: *Huntington's chorea in childhood.* Arch. Neurol. 9:244, 1963.

114. JOHNSON, R. T., AND JOHNSON, K. P.: Slow chronic virus infections of the nervous system, in Plum, F. (ed.): *Recent Advances in Neurology.* F. A. Davis Co., Philadelphia, 1969.

115. KARPATI, G., AND FRAME, B.: *Neuropsychiatric disorders in primary hyperparathyroidism.* Arch. Neurol. 10:387, 1964

116. KENYON, F. E., AND HARDY, S. M.: *A biochemical study of Huntington's chorea.* J. Neurol. Neurosurg. Psychiat. 26:123, 1963.

117. KESCHNER, M., BENDER, M. B., AND STRAUSS, I.: *Mental symptoms associated with brain tumor. Study of 530 verified cases.* J.A.M.A. 110:714, 1938.

118. KNEHR, C. A., AND BEARN, A. G.: *Psychological impairment in Wilson's disease.* J. Nerv. Ment. Dis. 124:251, 1956.

119. KOLODNY, A.: *The symptomatology of tumours of the temporal lobe.* Brain 51:385, 1928.

120. KRIGMAN, M. R., FELDMAN, R. G., AND BENSCH. K.: *Alzheimer's presenile dementia.* Lab. Invest. 14:381, 1965.

121. KURLAND, L. T., FARO, S. N., AND SIEDLER, H.: *Minamata disease.* World Neurol. 1:370, 1960.

122. LAFORA, G., AND GLUECK, B.: *Beitrag zur Histopathologie der myoklonischen Epilepsie.* Z. ges. Neur. Psychiat. 6:1, 1911.

123. LAMPERT, P., TOM, M. I., AND CUMINGS, J. N.: *Encephalopathy in Whipple's disease.* Neurology 12:65, 1962.

124. LEESE, S. M., POND, D. A., SHIELDS, J., AND RACE, R. R.: *A pedigree of Huntington's chorea, with a note on linkage data.* Ann. Eugen. 17:92, 1952.

125. LEHRER, G. M.: *Neuropsychiatric manifestations of hypercalcemia.* Arch. Neurol. Psychiat. 81:709, 1959.

126. LESSE, S., HOEFER, P. F. A., AND AUSTIN, J. H.: *The electroencephalogram in diffuse encephalopathies.* Arch. Neurol. Psychiat. 79:359, 1958.

127. LETEMENDIA, F., AND PAMPIGLIONE, G.: *Clinical and electroencephalographic observations in Alzheimer's disease.* J. Neurol. Neurosurg. Psychiat. 21:167, 1958.

128. LEVENTHAL, C. M., BARINGER, J. R., ARNASON, B. G., AND FISHER, C. M.: *A case of Marchiafava-Bignami disease with clinical recovery.* Trans. Amer. Neurol. Assn. 90:87, 1965.

129. LIDDELL, D. W.: *Investigations of EEG findings in presenile dementia.* J. Neurol. Neurosurg. Psychiat. 21:173, 1958.

130. LIN, J. P., GOODKIN, R., TONG, E. C. K., EPSTEIN, F. J., AND VINCIGUERRA, E.: *Radioiodinated serum albumin (RISA) cisternography in the diagnosis of incisural block and occult hydrocephalus.* Radiology 90:36, 1968.

131. LOCKE, S., MERRILL, J. P., AND TYLER, H. R.: *Neurological complications of uremia.* Arch. Int. Med. 108:519, 1961.

132. LORBER, J.: *Long-term follow-up of 100 children who recovered from tuberculous meningitis.* Pediatrics 28:778, 1961.

133. LUNDBORG, H.: *Der Erbang der progressiven Myoclonus-Epilepsie.* Z. ges. Neur. Psychiat. 9:353, 1912.

134. LUSE, S. A., AND SMITH, J. R.: *The ultrastructure of senile plaques.* Amer. J. Path. 44:553, 1964.

135. MAAS, O., AND PATERSON, A. S.: *Genetic and familial aspects of dystrophia myotonica.* Brain 66:55, 1943.

136. McGOVERN, G. P., MILLER, D. H., AND ROBERTSON, E.: *A mental syndrome associated with lung carcinoma.* Arch. Neurol. Psychiat. 81:341, 1959.

137. McMENEMEY, W. H.: *Alzheimer's disease: problems concerning its concept and nature.* Acta Neurol. Scand. 39:369, 1963.

138. McMENEMEY, W. H.: The dementias and progressive diseases of the basal ganglia, in Blackwood, W., et al. (eds.): *Greenfield's Neuropathology,* ed. 2. The Williams & Wilkins Co., Baltimore, 1966.

139. MAJTÉNY, K.: *Beiträge zur Pathologie der subakuten spongiösen Enzephalopathie.* Acta Neuropath. 4:491, 1965.

140. MALAMUD, N., AND COHEN, P.: *Unusual form of cerebellar ataxia with sex-linked inheritance.* Neurology 8:261, 1958.

141. MALAMUD, N., HIRANO, A., AND KURLAND, L. T.: *Pathoanatomic changes in amyotrophic lateral sclerosis on Guam—special reference to occurrence of neurofibrillary changes.* Arch. Neurol. 5:401, 1961.

142. MARIN, O., AND VIAL, J. D.: *Neuropathological and ultrastructural findings in two cases of subacute spongiform encephalopathy.* Acta Neuropath. 4:218, 1964.

143. MARKHAM, C. H., AND KNOX, J. W.: *Observations on Huntington's chorea in childhood.* J. Pediat. 67:46, 1965.

144. MAWDSLEY, C., AND FERGUSON, F. R.: *Neurological disease in boxers.* Lancet 2:795, 1963.

145. MAY, W. W.: *Creutzfeldt-Jakob disease. I. Survey of the literature and clinical diagnosis.* Acta Neurol. Scand. 44:1, 1968.

146. MAY, W. W., ITABASHI, H. H., AND DEJONG, R. N.: *Creutzfeldt-Jakob disease. II. Clinical, pathologic and genetic study of a family.* Arch. Neurol. 19:137, 1968.

147. MERRITT, H. H.: *A Textbook of Neurology,* ed. 4. Lea & Febiger, Philadelphia, 1967.

148. MESSERT, B., AND BAKER, N. H.: *Syndrome of progressive spastic ataxia and apraxia associated with occult hydrocephalus.* Neurology 16:440, 1966.

149. MEYER, A.: Intoxications, in Blackwood, W., et al. (eds.): *Greenfield's Neuropathology,* ed. 2. The Williams & Wilkins Co., Baltimore, 1966, Chap. 4.

150. MEYER, A.: The Hallervorden-Spatz syndrome, in Blackwood, W., et al. (eds.): *Greenfield's Neuropathology*, ed. 2. The Williams & Wilkins Co., Baltimore, 1966.

151. MEYER, A., LEIGH, D., AND BAGG, C. E.: *A rare presenile dementia associated with cortical blindness (Heidenhain's syndrome)*. J. Neurol. Neurosurg. Psychiat. 17:129, 1954.

152. MILLER, H., AND STERN, G.: *The long-term prognosis of severe head injury*. Lancet 1:225, 1965.

153. MOERSCH, F. P.: *Psychic manifestations in brain tumors*. Amer. J. Psychiat. 4:705, 1925.

154. MONIZ, E.: *Les tumeurs du corps calleux*. L'Encéphale 22:514, 1927.

155. MULDER, D. W.: Psychoses with brain tumors and other chronic neurologic disorders, in Arieti, S. (ed.): *American Handbook of Psychiatry*. Basic Books. New York, 1959, Chap. 55.

156. NEUMANN, M. A.: *Chronic progressive subcortical encephalopathy*—report of a case. J. Gerontol. 2:57, 1947.

157. NEUMANN, M. A., AND COHN, R.: *Incidence of Alzheimer's disease in a larger mental hospital*. Arch. Neurol. Psychiat. 69:615, 1953.

158. NEVIN, S., McMENEMEY, W. H., BEHRMAN, S., AND JONES, D. P.: *Subacute spongiform encephalopathy—A subacute form of encephalopathy attributable to vascular dysfunction (spongiform cerebral atrophy)*. Brain 83:519, 1960.

159. NICKEL, S. N., AND FRAME, B.: *Neurologic manifestations of myxedema*. Neurology 8:54, 1958.

160. NIEDERMEYER, E., ZELLWEGER, H., AND ALEXANDER, T.: *Central nervous system manifestations in myopathics*. Proceedings 8th International Congress of Neurology, Vienna, vol. 2, p. 293, 1965.

161. NOAD, K. B., AND LANCE, J. W.: *Familial myoclonic epilepsy and its association with cerebellar disturbance*. Brain 83:618, 1960.

162. O'CONNOR, J. F., AND MUSHER, D. M.: *Central nervous system involvement in systemic lupus erythematosus*. Arch. Neurol. 14:157, 1966.

163. OLIVECRONA, H., AND RIIVES, J.: *Arteriovenous aneurysms of the brain; their diagnosis and treatment*. Arch. Neurol. Psychiat. 59:567, 1948.

164. OLSZEWSKI, J.: *Subcortical arteriosclerotic encephalopathy*. World Neurol. 3:359, 1962.

165. OTO, Y.: Psychiatric studies on civilian head injuries, in Walker, A. E., Caveness, W. F., and Critchley, M. (eds.): *The Late Effects of Head Injury*. Charles C Thomas, Publisher, Springfield, Ill., 1969.

166. PALLIS, C. A., AND SPILLANE, J. D.: *A subacute progressive encephalopathy with mutism, hypokinesia, rigidity and myoclonus*. Quart. J. Med. 26:349, 1957.

167. PARKINSON, J.: An essay on the shaking palsy. Reprinted in Arch. Neurol. 20:441, 1969.

168. PARSONS, O. A., STEWART, K. D., AND ARENBERG, D.: *Impairment of abstracting ability in multiple sclerosis*. J. Nerv. Ment. Dis. 125:221, 1957.

169. PASKIND, H. A., AND STONE, T. T.: *Familial spastic paralysis.* Arch. Neurol. Psychiat. 30:481, 1933.

170. PATTERSON, R. M., BAGCHI, B. K., AND TEST, A.: *The prediction of Huntington's chorea, an electroencephalographic and genetic study.* Amer. J. Psychiat. 104:786, 1948.

171. PAULSON, G. W., KAPP, J., AND COOK, W.: *Dementia associated with bilateral carotid artery disease.* Geriatrics 21:159, 1966.

172. PAULSON, G. W., AND PERRINE, G., JR.: *Cerebral vascular disease in mental hospitals.* Transactions Sixth Conference on Cerebral Vascular Diseases. Grune & Stratton, New York, 1968.

173. PERLMUTTER, I.: *Subdural hematoma in older persons.* J.A.M.A. 176:212, 1961.

174. PIERCY, M.: Studies of the neurological basis of intellectual function, in Williams, D. (ed.) : *Modern Trends in Neurology.* Appleton-Century-Crofts, New York, 1967.

175. PLUM, F., AND POSNER, J. B.: *Diagnosis of Stupor and Coma.* F. A. Davis Co., Philadelphia, 1966.

176. PLUM, F., POSNER, J. B., AND HAIN, R. F.: *Delayed neurological deterioration after anoxia.* Arch. Int. Med. 110:18, 1962.

177. POLLOCK, M., AND HORNABROOK, R. W.: *The prevalence, natural history and dementia of Parkinson's disease.* Brain 89:429, 1966.

178. PRATT, R. T. C.: *The Genetics of Neurological Disorders.* Oxford monographs on medical genetics, Oxford University Press, New York, 1967.

179. RASKIN, N., AND EHRENBERG, R.: *Cerebral arteriosclerosis.* Amer. Pract. Digest Treatment 7:1095, 1956.

180. RASKIN, N., AND EHRENBERG, R.: *Senescence, senility and Alzheimer's disease.* Amer. J. Psychiat. 113:133, 1956.

181. REED, D., PLATO, C., ELIZAN, T., AND KURLAND, L. T.: *The ALS-Parkinsonism-dementia complex: A ten-year-follow-up on Guam.* Amer. J. Epidem. 83:54, 1966.

182. REFSUM, S., ENGESET, A., AND LÖNNUM, A.: *Pneumoencephalographic changes in dystrophia myotonica.* Acta Psychiat. Neurol. Scand. Suppl. 137:98, 1959.

183. REYNOLDS, E. H.: *Mental effects of anticonvulsants and folic acid metabolism.* Brain 91:197, 1968.

184. RICHARDSON, E. P., JR.: Progressive multifocal leukoencephalopathy, in Brain, R. L., and Norris, F. H., Jr. (eds.) : *Remote Effects of Cancer on the Nervous System.* Contemporary Neurology Symposia, Vol. I., Grune & Stratton, New York, 1965.

185. RICHARDSON, J. C., CHAMBERS, R. A., AND HEYWOOD, P. M.: *Encephalopathies of anoxia and hypoglycemia.* Arch. Neurol. 1:178, 1959.

186. RICHARDSON, M. E., AND BORNHOFEN, J. H.: *Early childhood cerebral lipidosis with prominent myoclonus.* Arch. Neurol. 18:34, 1968.

187. RIDDOCH, G.: *Progressive dementia, without headache or changes in the optic discs, due to tumours of the third ventricle.* Brain 59:225, 1936.

188. ROBINSON, K. C., KALLBERG, M. H., AND CROWLEY, M. F.: *Idiopathic hypoparathyroidism presenting as dementia.* Brit. Med. J. 2:1203, 1954.

189. ROSMAN, N. P., AND KAKULAS, B. A.: *Mental deficiency associated with muscular dystrophy. A neuropathological study.* Brain 89:769, 1966.

190. ROSS, A. T., AND REITAN, R. M.: *Intellectual and affective functions in multiple sclerosis.* Arch. Neurol. Psychiat. 13:663, 1955.

191. SAHS, A. L., AND JOYNT, R. J.: Meningitis, in Baker, A. B. (ed.) : *Clinical Neurology,* ed. 2. Hoeber-Harper, New York, 1962, Chap. 15.

192. SANDERS, V.: *Neurologic manifestations of myxedema.* New Eng. J. Med. 266:547 and 599, 1962.

193. SCHAUMBURG, H. H., AND SUZUKI, K. L.: *Non-specific familial presenile dementia.* J. Neurol. Neurosurg. Psychiat. 31:479, 1968.

194. SCHLESINGER, B.: *Mental changes in intracranial tumors and related problems.* Conf. Neurol. 10:225, 322, 1950.

195. SCHULMAN, S.: *Bilateral symmetrical degeneration of the thalamus.* J. Neuropath. Exp. Neurol. 15:208, 1956.

196. SCHWARZ, G. A., AND YANOFF, M.: *Lafora's disease—a distinct genetically determined form of Unverricht's syndrome.* Arch. Neurol. 12:172, 1965.

197. SCHWEDENBERG, T. H.: *Leukoencephalopathy following carbon monoxide asphyxia.* J. Neuropath. Exp. Neurol. 18:597, 1959.

198. SIEDLER, H., AND MALAMUD, N.: *Creutzfeldt-Jakob's disease.* J. Neuropath. Exp. Neurol. 22:381, 1963.

199. SILVERSTEIN, A.: *Occlusive disease of the carotid arteries.* Circulation 20:4, 1959.

200. SIM, M., AND SUSSMAN, I.: *Alzheimer's disease: Its natural history and differential diagnosis.* J. Nerv. Ment. Dis. 135:489, 1962.

201. SIMPSON, J. A.: *The neurological manifestations of idiopathic hypoparathyroidism.* Brain 75:76, 1952.

202. SJÖGREN, T.: *Klinische und erbbiologische Untersuchungen über die Heredoataxien.* Acta Psychiat. Kbh. Suppl. 27, 1943; quoted from Wilson, S. A. K.[256]

203. SJÖGREN, T., SJÖGREN, H., AND LINDGREN, A. G. H.: *Morbus Alzheimer and Morbus Pick. A genetic, clinical and pathoanatomical study.* Acta Psychiat. Neurol. Scand. Suppl. 82:1, 1952.

204. SMITH, A. D.: *Megaloblastic madness.* Brit. Med. J. 2:1840, 1960.

205. SONIAT, T. L. L.: *Psychiatric symptoms associated with intracranial neoplasms.* Amer. J. Psychiat. 108:19, 1951.

206. SPILLANE, J. D.: *Five boxers.* Brit. Med. J. 2:1205, 1962.

207. SPILLANE, J. D.: *Nervous and mental disorders in Cushing's syndrome.* Brain 74:72, 1951.

208. SPILLANE, J. D.: *Nutritional Disorders of the Nervous System.* Livingstone, Edinburgh, 1947.

209. SPROFKIN, B. E., AND SCIARRA, D.: *Korsakoff psychosis associated with cerebral tumors.* Neurology 2:427, 1952.

210. STEEGMAN, A. T.: *Anoxic encephalopathy and the cerebral circulation with reference to cardiovascular and respiratory disease.* Reports VII International Congress of Neurology, Rome, p. 197, 1961.

211. STEELE, J. C., RICHARDSON, J. C. AND OLSZEWSKI, J.: *Progressive supra-nuclear palsy.* Arch. Neurol. 10:333, 1964.

212. STENGEL, E.: *A study of the symptomatology and differential diagnosis of Alzheimer's disease and Pick's disease.* J. Ment. Sci. 89:1, 1943.

213. STERN, K.: *Severe dementia associated with bilateral symmetrical degeneration of the thalamus.* Brain 62:157, 1939.

214. STERN, M., AND ROBBINS, E. S.: *Psychoses in systemic lupus erythematosus.* Arch. Gen. Psychiat. 3:205, 1960.

215. STEVENS, H., AND FORSTER, F. M.: *Effect of carbon tetrachloride on the nervous system.* Arch. Neurol. Psychiat. 70:635, 1953.

216. STOUPEL, N., MONSEU, G., PARDOE, A., HEIMANN, R., AND MARTIN, J. J.: *Encephalitis with myoclonus in Whipple's disease.* J. Neurol. Neurosurg. Psychiat. 32:338, 1969.

217. STRACHAN, R. W.: *The natural history of Takayasu's arteriopathy.* Quart. J. Med. 33:57, 1964.

218. STRACHAN, R. W., AND HENDERSON, J. G.: *Dementia and folate deficiency.* Quart. J. Med. 60:189, 1967.

219. STRACHAN, R. W., AND HENDERSON, J. G.: *Psychiatric syndromes due to avitaminosis B_{12} with normal blood and bone marrow.* Quart. J. Med. 34:303, 1965.

220. STRICH, S. J.: The pathology of brain damage due to blunt head injuries, in Walker, A. E., Caveness, W. F., and Critchley, M. (eds.) : *The Late Effects of Head Injury.* Charles C Thomas, Publisher, Springfield, Ill., 1969.

221. STUTEVILLE, P., AND WELCH, K.: *Subdural hematoma in the elderly person.* J.A.M.A. 168:1445, 1958.

222. SUGAR, O.: *Central neurological complications of hypoparathyroidism.* Arch. Neurol. Psychiat. 70:86, 1953.

223. SWAIN, J. M.: *Electroencephalographic abnormalities in presenile atrophy.* Neurology 9:722, 1959.

224. SMYTH, G. E., AND STERN, K.: *Tumours of the thalamus—clinico-pathological study.* Brain 61:339, 1938.

225. TALLAND, G. A.: *Psychological studies of Korsakoff's psychosis. II. Perceptual functions.* J. Nerv. Ment. Dis. 127:197, 1958.

226. TALLAND, G. A.: *Psychological studies of Korsakoff's psychosis. III. Concept formation.* J. Nerv. Ment. Dis. 128:214, 1969.

227. TARKKANEN, J. V.: *Otogenic brain abscess.* Acta Otolaryng. Suppl. 185, 1963.

228. TAVERAS, J. M., AND WOOD, E. H.: *Diagnostic Neuroradiology.* The Williams & Wilkins Co., Baltimore, 1964.

229. TERRY, R. D.: *The fine structure of neurofibrillary tangles in Alzheimer's disease.* J. Neuropath. Exp. Neurol. 22:629, 1963.

230. TERRY, R. D., GONATAS, N. K., AND WEISS, M.: *Ultrastructural studies in Alzheimer's presenile dementia.* Amer. J. Path. 44:269, 1964.

231. THOMASEN, E.: *Myotonia.* Ejnar Munksgaard, Copenhagen, 1948.

232. TOMLINSON, B. E., BLESSED, G., AND ROTH, M.: *Observations on the brains of demented old people.* J. Neurol. Sci. 11:205, 1970.

233. TÖNNIS, W., SCHIEFER, W., AND WALTER, W.: *Signs and symptoms of supratentorial arteriovenous aneurysms.* J. Neurosurg. 15:471, 1958.

234. TOOLE, J. F., AND PATEL, A. N.: *Cerebrovascular Disorders.* McGraw-Hill Book Company, New York, 1967.

235. TRETHOWAN, W. H., AND COBB, S.: *Neuropsychiatric aspects of Cushing's syndrome.* Arch. Neurol. Psychiat. 67:283, 1952.

236. TYLER, H. R.: *Neurologic disorders in renal failure.* Amer. J. Med. 44:734, 1969.

237. TYNES, B. S., CRUTCHER, J. C., AND UTZ, J. P.: *Histoplasma meningitis.* Ann. Int. Med. 59:615, 1963.

238. UNVERRICHT, H.: *Die Myoclonie.* Franz Deuticke, Leipzig, 1891.

239. UNVERRICHT, H.: *Über familiäre Myoclonie.* Deut. Z. Nervenheilk. 7:32, 1895.

240. UTZ, J. P.: *Histoplasma and cryptococcus meningitis.* Res. Publ. Assn. Res. Nerv. Ment. Dis. 44:378, 1964.

241. VAN BUSKIRK, C.: Intracerebral vascular disease, in Baker, A. B. (ed.): *Clinical Neurology,* ed. 2. Hoeber-Harper, New York, 1962.

242. VAN DER ZWAN, A.: Late results from prolonged traumatic unconsciousness, in Walker, A. E., Caveness, W. F., and Critchley, M. (eds.): *The Late Effects of Head Injury.* Charles C Thomas, Publisher, Springfield, Ill., 1969.

243. VAN MANSFELT, J.: *Pick's Disease. A Syndrome of Lobar Cerebral Atrophy.* Enschede, 1954.

244. VERNON, M. L., PUCILLO, D. A., AND HAMILTON, R.: *Jacob-Creutzfeldt disease: Virus-like particles in two brain biopsies.* Fed. Proc. 29:286, 1970.

245. VICTOR, M.: Alcoholism, in Baker, A. B. (ed.): *Clinical Neurology.* Hoeber-Harper, New York, 1962, Chap. 22.

246. VICTOR, M., ADAMS, R. D., AND COLE, M.: *The acquired (non-Wilsonian) type of chronic hepatocerebral degeneration.* Medicine 44:345, 1965.

247. VICTOR, M., TALLAND, G. A., AND ADAMS, R. D.: *Psychological studies of Korsakoff's psychosis: I. General intellectual functions.* J. Nerv. Ment. Dis. 128:528, 1959.

248. WADIA, N., AND WILLIAMS, E.: *Behçet's syndrome with neurological complications.* Brain 80:59, 1957.

249. WAGGONER, R. W.: Brain syndromes associated with intracranial neoplasm, in Freedman, A. M., and Kaplan, H. I. (eds.): *Comprehensive Textbook of Psychiatry.* The Williams & Wilkins Co., Baltimore, 1967, Chap. 20.4.

250. WAGGONER, R. W., AND MALAMUD, N.: *Wilson's disease in the light of cerebral changes following ordinary acquired liver disorders.* J. Nerv. Ment. Dis. 96:410, 1942.

251. WALTHER-BÜEL, H.: *Die Psychiatrie der Hirngeschwülste.* Acta Neurochir. Suppl. 2, 1961.

252. WATSON, C. W., AND DENNY-BROWN, D.: *Myoclonus epilepsy as a symptom of diffuse neuronal disease.* Arch. Neurol. Psychiat. 70:151, 1953.

253. WILLANGER, R., THYGESEN, P., NIELSEN, R., AND PETERSON, O.: *Intellectual impairment and cerebral atrophy.* Danish Med. Bull. 15:65, 1968.

254. WILLIAMS, M., AND McGEE, T. F.: *Psychological study of carotid occlusion and endarterectomy.* Arch. Neurol. 10:293, 1964.

255. WILLIAMS, M., AND PENNYBACKER, J.: *Memory disturbances in third ventricle tumours.* J. Neurol. Neurosurg. Psychiat. 17:115, 1954.

256. WILSON, S. A. K.: *Neurology,* ed. 2, Butterworth and Co., Ltd., London, 1954.

257. WILSON, S. A. K.: *Progressive lenticular degeneration: A familial nervous disease associated with cirrhosis of the liver.* Brain 34:295, 1912.

258. WINKELMAN, N., AND BOOK, M. H.: *Asymptomatic extrapyramidal involvement in Pick's disease.* J. Neuropath. Exp. Neurol. 8:30, 1949.

259. WORDEN, D. K., AND VIGNOS, P. J.: *Intellectual function in childhood progressive muscular dystrophy.* Pediatrics 29:968, 1962.

260. ZU RHEIN, G. M., AND CHOU, S. M.: *Papova virus in progressive multifocal leukoencephalopathy.* Proc. Assn. Res. Nerv. Ment. Dis. 44:307, 1968.

Chapter 11

The Clinical Management
of the Patient with Dementia

Charles E. Wells, M.D.

Proper clinical management of the demented patient presents both diagnostic and therapeutic problems, not the least of which is the discouragement that the physician feels. Dementia is so common, particularly in the aged, and its precise etiology so rarely established that there is an ever present tendency to ascribe the dementia, with insufficient justification, to "cerebral arteriosclerosis" or, with even less justification, to "old age." Were there a readily available therapeutic regimen promising dramatic symptom relief, then at least therapeutic pessimism might not be joined to the diagnostic dilemma. Unfortunately, save for the few dementias of specific known cause and treatment, there are no therapeutic measures that assure clinical improvement. Thus neither the patient nor the physician can confront the situation with any realistic degree of optimism.

As patients with dementia are studied with increasing thoroughness, more treatable cases of dementia are being uncovered. It is essential, therefore, that the patient with a treatable disease not be overlooked. The physician must train himself to suspect dementia even on the basis of inadequate evidence. Once the question of dementia is raised, he uses the history and mental status evaluation to test this possibility. Adding to this the observations obtained from general physical and neurological examinations, he makes hypotheses as to the nature of the disorder and the site of involvement. These hypotheses are tested by further diagnostic studies, so that he arrives at a firm diagnosis and a rational process of treatment. The physician must thus assimilate a systematic plan for patient care by which he can: (1) prove or disprove the presence of dementia; (2) arrive at a correct diagnosis of its cause; and (3) treat the patient by the best means available.

PATIENT EVALUATION

History

When the patient comes to the physician complaining of the classic symptoms of organic brain disease as outlined in the A.P.A.'s *Diagnostic and Statistical Manual*[3] (loss of memory, inability to calculate, disorientation, for example), only a little perspicacity is required to suspect dementia and to confirm the diagnosis. Fortunately from the patient's point of view, though perhaps not from the physician's, the classic symptoms and signs of dementia may be rather late-stage events, and the initial events, when the patient is most amenable to treatment, may prove hazy and evanescent.[39] In the initial evaluation of the patient, three situations should particularly signal the diagnostic possibility of dementia:

1. The physician is suspicious if the patient presents multiple physical complaints that fit into no discernible pattern of physical disease. He is particularly suspicious if these complaints do not fit into the previous life style of the individual.

2. The physician is suspicious if a patient presents a variety of "psychiatric" symptoms, such as depression, anxiety, and irritability. He is even more suspicious when the symptoms fit into no specific functional diagnostic category and when the patient has no history of previous emotional problems.

3. The physician is suspicious if the patient presents a story that remains vague and unclear to the examiner even after a lengthy and sympathetic hearing. This occurs with many illnesses, but the possibility of dementia is always raised by its occurrence.

When the patient's symptoms are centered upon emotional experiences, two tendencies must particularly be guarded against. The first tendency is to regard, in an almost automatic fashion, all mental dysfunction in the young as functional or nonorganic in origin, thereby neglecting the possibility of organic cerebral disease in younger patients; the converse tendency is to regard all mental symptoms presenting in old age as due to cerebral deterioration. Both Busse[10] and Roth[31] have emphasized the frequency of nonorganic mental disorders, particularly depressive illness, in the aged and their excellent prognosis with appropriate treatment.

Once dementia is suspected, there are a number of historical factors to be investigated. A precise description of the presenting symptoms is essential, if the patient or his associates can provide it. Has there been memory loss? Has there been difficulty concentrating, dealing with complex materials, keeping facts and schedules in order? Do the complaints lie largely within the cognitive and intellectual sphere, or are they largely affectual in nature? The mode of onset and progression is of special importance in suggesting the etiology of the disorder. Abruptness of onset and a stuttering course are characteristic of vascular disease, as are the appearance and resolution of focal neurological symptoms and signs; such a progression is not foreign, however, to the primary cerebral degenerative processes.[37] Have there been headaches, changes in level of consciousness, or epileptic seizures? A history of even slight cranial trauma may prove important. With the increasingly generalized use of sedatives, tranquilizers, and antidepressant medications, a thorough history of the patient's use of drugs, including alcohol, is essential. Is there a history of anemia? Has the patient experienced malaise, loss of energy, anorexia, or weight loss—all of which might suggest the presence of occult malignant disease? Has there been fever, or is there a history of chronic infectious processes? Are there symptoms that suggest Parkinson's disease?

The patient must also be questioned about specific symptoms that suggest focal cerebral dysfunction. Have there been language difficulties? Has he had difficulty understanding or reading words? Has he forgotten "how to do" things? Is there difficulty attending to and following instructions? Is there loss of recent memory, trouble recognizing people and objects? Has neglect of one side of the body or one half of space been noted? Are there symptoms of focal weakness or sensory loss?

Since dementia occurs with many systemic diseases,[17] a thorough review of systems is essential. Are there symptoms or a history of syphilis? Does dyspnea, cough, or sputum production suggest chronic pulmonary disease? Does hematuria, scant urine, or edema point toward chronic renal dysfunction? Is there jaundice, itching, dark urine, or light stools compatible with liver dysfunction? Do changes in habitus, heat and cold tolerance, and hair texture and distribution suggest an endocrinological disorder?

Mental Status Evaluation

Often the presence of dementia can be established by a simple psychiatric examination demonstrating loss of memory for recent events, spatial and temporal disorientation, and generally diminished intellectual capacities; or its presence can safely be disallowed by a thoroughgoing psychiatric examination that establishes none of the features of organic brain disease. Commonly, however, the suspicion of organic brain dysfunction is not easily put to rest. The person suspected of dementia is often elderly when some decline in mental capacity is accepted as normal.[38] In younger individuals, massive employment of defenses such as denial and repression may suggest a hysterical memory loss and hide the underlying organic process.[22] A systematic assay of the patient's mental status usually provides the physician some certainty in his diagnosis.

A significant portion of the mental status examination is, in fact, performed in the history-taking process. In general, this establishes the level and competence of the patient's mentative capacities over a wide range of functions, including recent and remote memory, affect, and capacity for logical thought. The more formal portions of the mental status examination (described in the following paragraphs) are useful, however: (1) to establish with more certainty the presence of dementia, which is suspected but not proved on the basis of the history; (2) to establish a quantitative baseline of function from which further progression or regression can be measured; (3) to delineate specific mentative dysfunctions (particularly amnestic, agnosic, apractic, aphasic features) [18] that have focal significance. A schema for the systematic mental status evaluation is outlined in Table 1; this follows in large part the examination suggested by McDowell and Wolff.[24]

APPEARANCE AND BEHAVIOR. How does the patient present himself? Is he clean, neatly dressed, and appropriately groomed, or is he perhaps unclean with clothing in disarray? Does he look older or younger than his years? Does his appearance reflect his position in the world? Is he alert and responsive or dull and apathetic? Is he drowsy and unable to attend to the questioner? Are his movements slow and sparse, or is he tremulous, changing positions frequently, wringing his hands, or unable to sit for the examination? Is he friendly, cooperative, distant, or truculent? Can he attend to the examination, or does his mind frequently wander from the point?

ORIENTATION. Unless the patient's orientation is established without question from the history, it must be proved by direct questioning. Does the patient

Table I. Mental status examinations

Apperance and behavior
Orientation
Speech
Mood
Memory
General intellectual evaluation
Special preoccupations and experiences
Understanding

know his name, where he is, the time of day, the day of the week, the date, the year, the season?

SPEECH. Is there a paucity of speech, or is the patient loquacious? Are words clearly pronounced? Are there defects in sentence structure? Does he misuse words, seem to have trouble finding words, talk "around" a missing word, or use nonexistent words? Is there perseveration or blocking of speech? Is his speech relevant to the question asked, and does the flow of talk follow a logical course?

MOOD. Although mood can often be inferred from the general tenor of the conversation, it should be delineated by specific questions. "How are your spirits?" "Are you afraid, fearful, anxious?" If the patient's mood is elevated, is it inappropriate? If his mood is sad, does he have thoughts, plans, or fears of suicide?

MEMORY. Several categories of memory must be tested.[18]

Immediate Recall. This is generally measured by asking the patient to repeat digits after the examiner, beginning with three and increasing the number of digits until the patient begins to fail. The patient is tested first for recall of digits to be repeated just as the examiner said them; then he is asked to repeat them backward. In general, most patients can repeat at least six digits forward and four backward without significant difficulty.

The patient may also be asked to repeat three unrelated words immediately and then after 5 minutes.

Recent Memory. The patient is asked to tell the examiner of events in his immediate past. How did he get to the doctor's office? If hospitalized, for how long? What did he eat last? What are the names of doctors, nurses, and family who have attended him?

Remote Memory. Can the patient tell the examiner the date of his birth, parents' names, schools attended and their order, jobs held and their sequence, date of marriage, names of children?

General Grasp and Recall. The patient is given a series of increasingly complex tasks to perform: "Raise your right arm." "Put your left index finger on your nose." "Put your right index finger on your left eye." "Put your right index finger on your left ear and your left index finger on your right eye." Frequently the examiner will note the patient's performance to falter as the tasks grow more difficult.

The examiner may read the following story, asking the patient to recount its details immediately afterward: "A cowboy from Arizona went to San Francisco with his dog, which he left with a friend while he purchased a new suit of clothes. Dressed finely, he went back to the dog, whistled to him, called him by name, and patted him. But the dog would have nothing to do with him in his new hat and coat, but gave a mournful howl. Coaxing was of no effect, so the cowboy went away and donned his old garments whereupon the dog immediately showed his wild joy on seeing his master." The patient's version may be recorded and its accuracy verified.

GENERAL INTELLECTUAL EVALUATION. The patient's responses to this portion of the examination will, of course, depend to a large extent upon his past experience. Thus a better performance is expected from a college graduate than from one who dropped out of school in the eighth grade. In the very sophisticated patient, a general intellectual evaluation can often best be obtained through the general history. When there is deterioration, however, or when the patient has a limited background, specific questions may be valuable.

General Information. "Who is President of the United States?" "Name the Presidents going backward as far as you can recall." "Who is the Vice-President, Governor of your state, Senators who represent your state in Congress?" "Name five of the largest cities in the United States." "Name the states that border on your home state." "Give an explanation of the seasons of the year."

Calculations. "Subtract 7 from 100, then continue subtracting 7 from each sum obtained." "Compute 2×3, 5×8, 9×12, 12×13."

Can the patient perform the multiplication tables? "If eggs are $1.20 per dozen, what would be the cost of three eggs?"

Discrimination and Judgment. Can the patient describe the difference or similarity between a child and a dwarf, a tree and a bush, a river and a canal, a lie and a mistake, a coat and a dress? Can he explain the difference between idleness and laziness, poverty and misery, character and reputation? Can he interpret proverbs appropriately, or does he describe their meaning in concrete terms?

Ask the patient to answer the following questions: (1) "If you drove into an unfamiliar city seeking to find a friend living there, how would you go about reaching him?" (2) "If you got into your automobile one morning planning to go to work but found the car would not start, how would you handle the situation?"

Ask the patient to estimate the length of a minute without regarding a watch. Normally a person estimates between 50 and 70 seconds. After he has made the estimate, ask the patient how he performed this task, for most individuals count slowly to 60 in order to give a correct response.

214

SPECIAL PREOCCUPATIONS AND EXPERIENCES. *Preoccupations.* Are there feelings, thoughts, worries, or concerns that stay on the patient's mind that he cannot stop thinking about?

Hallucinations. The examiner must determine if the patient has visual, olfactory, auditory, or tactile hallucinations. Questions that may elicit these symptoms are: "Do you see or hear things that you know aren't there?" "Have you ever had visions?" "Do you hear noises or voices or see objects that others appear unaware of?"

Illusions. Does the patient misinterpret sensory stimuli; for example, is a fluttering curtain misinterpreted as someone climbing through the window, are specks of dirt misinterpreted as small insects, is a shadow upon the wall misinterpreted as an animal?

Delusions. Does the patient possess false beliefs such as extreme poverty or wealth, wickedness or guilt, health or disease, unusual bodily changes, persecutions or dangers? Some appropriate questions to elicit these beliefs are: "Have people treated you strangely?" "Do you feel people take undue notice of you?" "Has anyone attempted to hurt or injure you?" "Do you believe outside forces such as electricity or television influence your mind or body?" "Do you seem to be under outside control?"

Obsessions, Compulsions, Phobias, and Rituals. "Do you have habits that bother you?" "Do you have special ways of doing things, so that it disturbs you if you are not able to do them in this fashion?" "Do you have recurrent thoughts or ideas that you cannot get out of your mind?" "Do you feel compelled to perform certain acts that seem to you to have no reason?"

UNDERSTANDING. To what extent does the patient comprehend his current situation and recognize his difficulties? Does he know that he is ill? Does he feel that all of this attention is unnecessary? Does he feel that nothing is wrong with him and that he should be elsewhere? Does he understand why he is being examined?

Such is the makeup of a thorough mental status evaluation. It is valuable not only to determine whether or not a patient has evidence of organic mental dysfunction but also to establish a level of functioning with precision, so that future changes can be measured against it.

Physical Examination

The patient suspected of having dementia requires not only a thorough psychiatric examination but a complete medical and neurological evaluation as well. The general medical evaluation is directed particularly at uncovering evidence of these systemic disorders that might account for the dementia.[17] Does the patient have fever suggesting an infectious process? Is the blood pressure elevated so that cerebral vascular disease might be suspected? Is the pulse irregular, a common finding with cerebral embolism? Does examination of the skin suggest anemia, jaundice, polycythemia, endocrine dysfunction, malnutrition? Does the breath smell of uremia or alcohol? Are the lymph nodes enlarged such as might be found with a chronic granulomatous process or Hodgkin's disease?

The cardiovascular system is thoroughly evaluated for evidence of cardiac enlargement, venous engorgement, and pulmonary and peripheral edema. The physician evaluates pulmonary function also, particularly observing the patient for dyspnea, cyanosis, pulmonary congestion, and impaired respiratory movements. The abdomen is palpated for evidence of an enlarged or nodular liver and of splenic or renal enlargement. The patient's habitus, hair texture, hair distribution, and skin texture are observed particularly for evidence of endocrinological disorder.

Neurological Examination

A careful, thorough neurological examination is required for each subject suspected of dementia. No attempt is made here to replicate directions for such detailed examinations as are covered in the standard neurological texts. Rather the specific aims of the neurological examination in dementia will be enumerated and particular features of the examination emphasized.

When dementia is suspected, the neurological examination seeks to establish one of three positions: (1) The neurological examination reveals clear evidence of focal, circumscribed brain disease accounting for the patient's symptoms. (2) The neurological examination reveals clear evidence of diffuse, bilateral brain dysfunction accounting for the patient's symptoms. (3) The neurological examination reveals no evidence of neurological dysfunction.

The "routine" neurological examination as described in most textbooks is designed to establish the first or last position. This portion of the evaluation will not be considered further here, save for the observation that its expert and detailed accomplishment is required for each patient.

Evidence for diffuse brain dysfunction is generally more subtle and harder to come by, as Paulson[30] has emphasized. At the outset attention is directed toward the patient's level of consciousness, attentiveness to the examiner, comprehension, and performance of requested tasks. Note is also made of the patient's facial expressions, quality of speech, body posture, respiratory rhythm, and gait. Specific signs of diffuse brain dysfunction sought include: persistence of glabella-tap response, corneomandibular reflex, sucking reflex, snout reflex, palmomental reflex, grasp reflex, and toe grasp reflex. While these signs may occasionally have focal import, they are much more likely to reflect diffuse brain dysfunction. Paratonic rigidity, motor perseveration, and motor impersistence are other features pointing toward diffuse disease.

DIAGNOSTIC CONCLUSIONS AND FURTHER STUDIES

On the basis of the history plus the examinations detailed above, the physician usually reaches one of several possible tentative conclusions that dictate further specific diagnostic studies:

1. The patient has no dementia but rather a functional disorder for which psychiatric treatment is indicated.

2. The patient has dementia secondary to a focal cerebral lesion whose nature must be elucidated.

3. The patient may have dementia, but this is not definite. If so, the dementia is probably secondary to diffuse cerebral dysfunction.

4. The patient has dementia, probably secondary to diffuse cerebral dysfunction.

The first two conclusions require relatively little consideration here; the last two require detailed treatment.

The Patient with a Functional Disorder

The physician reaches this conclusion with various degrees of certainty. If the absence of dementia is without doubt, and if the precise psychiatric diagnosis is established, then the physician proceeds at once either to initiate psychiatric therapy himself or to refer the patient to a psychiatrist for appropriate treatment.

If this conclusion appears justified, but not with certainty, then further diagnostic studies are appropriate to confirm the impression. Psychological testing is particularly useful in this instance, because these procedures may both show a lack of evidence of organic brain dysfunction and reveal definite evidence of a specific functional disorder. Sometimes further studies—especially skull x-rays, brain scan, and electroencephalogram (EEG) —may be added in an attempt to adduce further evidence that there is no organic cerebral disease, but all these procedures may remain normal even with significant underlying brain disease.

The Patient with Dementia Due to a Focal Cerebral Lesion

This conclusion has usually been reached because: (1) The history and mental status examination have revealed a defect (for example, aphasia) likely due to dysfunction within a limited area of brain; or (2) the neurological examination indicates a focal cerebral lesion. In either event, the patient will be admitted to the hospital for an evaluation that usually follows predictable lines. Though the exact makeup and order of diagnostic tests differ from patient to patient, skull x-ray studies, EEG, examination of cerebrospinal fluid, and brain scan usually constitute the initial procedures, followed by cerebral angiography or air encephalography or both. These procedures aim to demonstrate a treatable focal lesion. When such a lesion is revealed (as with a subdural hematoma), surgical treatment is generally indicated. When untreatable focal lesions (such as brain infarction) are revealed, therapy must be largely symptomatic.

The Patient with Possible or Proved Dementia, Probably Due to Diffuse Cerebral Disease

When the physician reaches these conclusions, an extensive diagnostic evaluation is needed.

PSYCHOLOGICAL TESTING. When the diagnosis of dementia has not been established, the physician frequently turns first to the psychologist for assistance. Even when dementia has been confirmed by the mental status examination, however, the psychologist may be called upon for help in determining the exact extent and severity of the mentative incapacity. Many of the psychological tests and measures have been discussed.[19] The psychologist is likely to prove most useful to the physician: (1) when the physician states precisely to the psychologist the problem with which he is seeking assistance; and (2) when the physician is familiar enough with the psychological testing procedures that he is personally able to evaluate and criticize the test results.

Certain observations—a discrepancy between verbal and performance I.Q.'s on the Wechsler Adult Intelligence Scale (WAIS); an abnormal "deterioration index" on the WAIS; poor reproduction of the Bender Visual Motor Gestalt Test; poverty of production, poor percepts, and failure to see movement on the Rorschach Test; poor performance on the Trailmaking Test—suggest individually the presence of organic brain dysfunction. When these psychological dysfunctions occur in a constellation, the probability that the patient has organic brain disease is increased.

Psychological testing is further valuable in setting a baseline from which the progression or resolution of the disease process may be followed and in evaluating residual function so that realistic treatment and rehabilitation plans can be made.[19] Psychological testing may also be useful in pointing away from an organic and toward a functional etiology, as for example in the elderly individual with psychotic depression who presents many superficial features of dementia.

BASIC EVALUATION PROCEDURES. Once dementia is established and diffuse brain disease is presumed, a search for the cause must be instituted. In most instances the patient should be admitted to the hospital for further medical and neurological diagnostic procedures. Outpatient examination alone for such serious disorders invites a slighting evaluation and the acceptance of superficial diagnostic explanations. In the young or middle-aged patient presenting with dementia, hospitalization would be generally considered a necessity. At a more advanced age, however, such scrupulous attention to detail might not generally be forthcoming; the patient might rather by default be assigned a diagnosis of cerebral vascular disease or senile dementia. While these are frequent causes of dementia in old age, they are nevertheless discreet entities and should not be "wastebasket" diagnoses. Eschewing facile diagnoses, therefore, almost every patient presenting with dementia should be

Table 2. Basic laboratory procedures for evaluation of dementia of unknown cause

Test	Rationale—The Test May Demonstrate . . .
Chest x ray	Infectious process, primary or metastatic tumor, chronic lung disease
Skull x ray	Unsuspected focal lesion, pineal shift, evidence of increased intracranial pressure, disordered calcium metabolism
Electroencephalogram	Unsuspected focal lesion or diffuse cerebral dysfunction
Brain scan	Unsuspected focal lesion
Electrocardiogram	Arrhythmia, evidence of recent or remote myocardial infarction
Urinalysis	Renal disease, hepatic disease
Schilling test	Impaired vitamin B_{12} absorption
Blood tests	
complete blood count	Anemia (megaloblastic or hypochromic), infection
serological test for syphilis (STS)	Syphilis
drug levels (barbiturates, bromides, etc.)	Drug intoxication
electrolytes (sodium potassium, chloride, carbon dioxide, calcium)	Pulmonary dysfunction, renal dysfunction, endocrine dysfunction
urea nitrogen	Renal dysfunction
liver function tests (bilirubin, enzymes, ammonia if available)	Hepatic dysfunction
protein bound iodine	Thyroid dysfunction
Cerebrospinal fluid pressure, protein, cells, sugar (if cells are increased), STS	Nature of intracranial disease (degeneration, chronic infection, syphilis, etc.).

admitted to the hospital for thorough medical, neurological, and psychiatric evaluation.

Table 2 lists the basic laboratory procedures that should be employed in most patients admitted for diagnosis of dementia thought due to diffuse brain disease, along with the rationale for the suggested tests. Not every test is required in every patient. For example, if the history and physical examination suggest vitamin B_{12} deficiency, then the diagnosis might be established by demonstration of a megaloblastic anemia plus a positive Schilling test demonstrating impaired absorption of vitamin B_{12}. When the history and physical examination do not point toward a specific cause for the presenting dementia, however, the procedures listed in Table 2 serve as a useful guide for excluding most of the treatable causes. Rarely is a less complete evaluation acceptable.

DIFFERENTIAL DIAGNOSIS AND SPECIFIC TREATMENT

The diagnostic process outlined above is designed particularly to reveal causes of dementia for which specific treatments are available. In this section discrete disorders are discussed, with attention to specific diagnostic and treatment requirements.

Vitamin B_{12} Deficiency

Vitamin B_{12} (cyanocobalamin) deficiency is often associated with mentative difficulties. The cerebral dysfunction does not correlate well with the degree of anemia. Thus while the presence of a megaloblastic anemia in a demented patient strongly suggests vitamin B_{12} deficiency, the absence of anemia does not rule against it.

Cyanocobalamin absorption is usually best evaluated by the Schilling test. In this procedure, a small quantity of Co^{57}-labeled cyanocobalamin is given orally along with a large parenteral dose of the unlabeled vitamin; urinary excretion of the labeled vitamin is measured for a 24-hour period. In the normal individual 7 per cent or more of the ingested labeled vitamin is excreted in the 24-hour urine sample; in the individual with deficient absorption, less than 2 per cent usually appears in the urine. If less than 7 per cent is excreted in the 24-hour urine, the test should be repeated with intrinsic factor.

The patient with cerebral dysfunction secondary to vitamin B_{12} deficiency is treated with daily injections of 100 to 200 μg. of vitamin B_{12} for 1 to 2 weeks, thereafter on a monthly basis. Restitution of normal function may not occur if treatment is delayed too long.

Syphilis

General paresis, a frequent cause of dementia only a few years ago, is now uncommon, so much so that there is danger of its being overlooked. In general paresis, both blood and cerebrospinal fluid reagin tests are usually strongly positive. In rare cases, however, the spinal fluid reagin test is positive when the blood is negative. A negative blood reaction thus does not rule out central nervous system syphilis. In general paresis there are usually other cerebrospinal fluid abnormalities as well, with increase in cells and protein and a first zone gold curve being usual.[27]

In the past few years, several studies have suggested that ocular syphilis may occur as a progressive disorder when blood and spinal fluid reagin tests are negative, the diagnosis being established by a positive Fluorescent Treponemal Antibody-Absorption (FTA–ABS) blood test.[35, 36] To date, convincing examples of clinically progressive general paresis with negative blood and cerebrospinal fluid reagin tests and positive FTA–ABS blood test responding to appropriate antisyphilitic treatment have not been reported. In the rare patient with progressive dementia, a history of untreated syphilis, and negative reagin tests, the FTA–ABS test on blood should be employed.[28]

General paresis is treated with a total of 20 to 25 million units of penicillin given in equal daily doses over a 10- to 14-day period.

Chronic Drug Intoxication

Symptoms and signs of dementia are a common byproduct of excessive prolonged use of drugs, particularly bromides, barbiturates, and tranquilizers. The diagnosis is suspected with a history of chronic drug ingestion and is proved with the demonstration of elevated blood levels of the specific agent. It can be strongly suspected without confirmatory blood levels when the patient's dementia shows remarkable improvement without specific treatment during a period of hospitalization.

There is some question as to whether prolonged excessive use of centrally acting drugs can produce cerebral atrophy. Certainly cerebral atrophy can be demonstrated in some patients who chronically abuse drugs, but it cannot be proved that the atrophy is due to the drugs. In patients with proved cerebral atrophy and a history of excessive drug use, improvement in mentation may follow discontinuance of the drugs.[20]

Chronic Alcoholism

Much that was said for chronic drug intoxication is true for the dementia accompanying chronic alcoholism. This situation is perhaps even more complex because of the vitamin deficiency, malnutrition, and multiple systemic disorders often complicating the alcoholism. Even when the dementia is long-standing and profound, remarkable improvement may occur with abstinence from alcohol and the institution of a nutritious diet.[40]

Thyroid Disease

Both hypothyroidism and hyperthyroidism are accompanied by symptoms and signs of dementia.[41] In general, the dysfunction is greatest in the hypothyroid patient in whom depression plus cognitive and intellectual deficits may be prominent. The severity of the mental dysfunction can be correlated roughly with the severity of thyroid dysfunction.

With even mild degrees of thyroid dysfunction, changes in cerebration can be demonstrated. The diagnosis of thyroid disease is usually suspected on the basis of the physical examination and confirmed by laboratory studies. The blood protein bound iodine (PBI) determination (normal usually between 3.5 and 8 μg. per 100 ml.) is probably the most readily available and most reliable of the tests commonly used to evaluate thyroid function. Even mild deviations from the normal should suggest that thyroid dysfunction is contributing to the mental trouble and lead to appropriate treatment. The radioactive iodine uptake (RAI) test may supplement or confirm the PBI.

The treatment of hyperthyroidism is a complex topic which will not be dealt with here. Treatment for hypothyroidism is generally with desiccated thyroid, 0.1 to 0.2 gm. daily at the outset, with the dose being regulated later on the basis of clinical response. In older patients, smaller amounts of thyroid are generally employed initially.

Cushing's Syndrome

Mental changes are common in this disorder. The diagnosis is usually suspected on the basis of the patient's habitus, plus skin changes and alteration in hair texture and distribution. The diagnosis is confirmed by the demonstration of excessive excretion of urinary glucocorticoids and of elevated plasma corticosteroids. For further details concerning the diagnosis and treatment of Cushing's syndrome, the reader is referred to textbooks of endocrinology.

Chronic Pulmonary, Hepatic, and Renal Disease

Dementia occurs in chronic lung, liver, and kidney disease. In each disorder, however, the appearance of dementia is determined by multiple factors and cannot be related to a single feature of the disease or to a single laboratory abnormality. In general, dementia occurs only in severe lung, liver, or kidney disease with severe metabolic derangement. Individual susceptibility to the development of cerebral symptoms is marked. Treatment here is directed toward the primary disease.

Parkinson's Disease

Dementia, along with depression, is a frequent accompaniment of Parkinson's disease. In general, however, the disturbance in motility has been so serious an impediment to normal function that it has overshadowed the mental dysfunction. The introduction of L-dopa treatment for the disordered motility has led to a reassessment of this problem. When studied by psychological methods, intellectual impairment can be demonstrated frequently in patients with Parkinson's disease, and improvement in intellectual function can be demonstrated when the patient is treated with appropriate amounts of L-dopa.[25]

Cryptococcal Meningitis

Cryptococcal meningitis is another cause of dementia that can be treated effectively. Since the usual diagnostic methods (India-ink preparations and cerebrospinal fluid culture) are not completely reliable, how far should the physician go to rule out this treatable disorder? Although cryptococcal meningitis has been reported in the absence of cerebrospinal fluid pleocytosis,[12] It seems unlikely that dementia could result from cryptococcal meningitis if the patient is afebrile, has normal cells and sugar in the cerebrospinal fluid, and has no condition that would predispose to infection (such as Hodgkin's disease or lupus erythematosus). Should the demented patient have fever or a condition predisposing to infection, a normal cerebrospinal fluid examination and a negative India-ink preparation do not rule out cryptococcal disease, and a latex slide agglutination test for specific cryptococcal antigen or a complement fixation test for cryptococcal polysaccharide should be performed.[6, 15] Treatment with intravenous amphotericin B over long periods has proved quite effective.

Cerebral Arteriosclerosis

Cerebral arteriosclerosis or cerebral vascular disease is probably the most common diagnosis assigned to the patient with dementia, especially if the patient is elderly. The diagnosis is often incorrect, and its facile application results in failure to identify cases of dementia which are treatable. Cerebral vascular disease seldom if ever causes the progressive deterioration of mentative function along with neurological signs of diffuse brain disease seen in Alzheimer's disease and senile dementia. Dementia due to cerebral vascular disease is almost always manifested by a stuttering course and by symptoms and signs of focal cerebral damage.[14] Nevertheless, even without an episodic course and without transient signs of focal dysfunction, dementia is often ascribed to cerebral vascular disease because there is evidence for peripheral atherosclerosis, though it has been known for years that the cerebral vessels do not predictably reflect the degree of atherosclerosis seen in peripheral and retinal vessels.[2] Cerebral vascular disease should never be accepted as the "cause" of dementia without a history of clear exacerbations and remissions punctuating the downhill clinical course and without previous history or present signs of focal brain damage.

FURTHER DIAGNOSTIC STUDIES

Should the diagnostic studies suggested in Table 2 and further elaborated in the text fail to establish an etiology for the dementia—and this would not be uncommon—four further diagnostic procedures are usually considered—serial brain scan after subarachnoid radioactive iodinated serum albumin (RISA) injections, cerebral arteriography, cerebral air studies, and brain biopsy.[26] Differences of opinion exist as to whether any or all these measures should be employed in the patient whose dementia remains unexplained.

The RISA scan is expensive and time consuming but of little danger or discomfort to the patient. In this group its diagnostic yield is likely to be low, but when it is positive (i.e., when occult hydrocephalus with malabsorption of cerebrospinal fluid is demonstrated) a treatable condition has been uncovered. Thus it should be employed in almost every instance of progressive dementia for which no other cause can be established.

Cerebral arteriography is a widely employed diagnostic procedure carrying with it a significant morbidity that is increased in the presence of underlying vascular disease. It is of particular value in focal cerebral disease. Because of its morbidity and specific utility in the demonstration of focal but not diffuse brain lesions, it should be employed only in selected cases of unexplained dementia.

Air studies (pneumoencephalography and ventriculography) are widely employed diagnostically and also result in significant morbidity but in a negligible mortality. They reveal both focal and diffuse brain lesions, however, and they permit definitive diagnosis of occult hydrocephalus and cerebral atrophy. Pneumoencephalography should be employed in almost every patient whose dementia remains unexplained after complete preliminary studies. The exceptions are the patient whose dementia is so longstanding as to make any treatment unlikely to succeed and the patient whose debility suggests his inability to tolerate the procedure with safety.

The possibility of a cerebral biopsy for diagnostic purposes is often raised. While the procedure is not particularly dangerous, it does require the neurosurgical opening of the skull—a situation not to be lightly regarded by physician or patient. Furthermore, the utility of the cerebral biopsy to either physician or patient is limited. In 15 patients with presenile dementia subjected to cerebral biopsy, 7 revealed changes of Alzheimer's disease and 8 revealed nonspecific changes.[16] In another study of 59 patients with presenile dementia evaluated by cerebral biopsy, the histological diagnoses were: nonspecific in 17 cases, consistent with Alzheimer's disease in 34, combined Alzheimer's and Pick's in 1, possible Pick's disease in 2, arteriopathic cerebral atrophy in 2, subacute spongiform encephalopathy in 1, and chronic meningoencephalitis in 2.[33] In these two studies therefore, from the standpoint of clinical management, brain biopsy did little other than confirm the presence of some sort of underlying brain disease whose presence has presumably already been proved by other methods. Thus diagnostic cerebral biopsy should rarely be employed in clinical evaluation of dementia, though it might form an essential part of research in this area.

NONSPECIFIC TREATMENT

Close attention to diagnostic detail is essential if we are to identify each example of dementia amenable to treatment before irreversible brain damage has occurred—but the yield will be low and the results disappointing. At the present stage of our knowledge, most patients with dementia will not have a precise cause identified, or if a specific diagnosis is established, there will be no remedy available. Most often then, the damage will proceed despite all the physician's efforts. This situation of apparent hopelessness is ripe for the rejection of the patient by the physician and by the family. We are apt to forget that it is in just such situations where there is no specific treatment that the treatment of the patient himself becomes most important. It is in just such "hopeless" situations where the acts and powers of the physician, as opposed to the effects of his medicines, become of greatest value. Here the psychiatric evaluation of the patient and the psychiatric aspects of his care become paramount.

Even though we accept as the physician's function always to offer comfort and succor, the behavior of the demented patient often makes it seem that comfort is not wanted, needed, or possible. Frequently the patient appears oblivious to his plight, untroubled by his failures, and unaffected by his deterioration. While such loss of contact with reality does occur in the most profound stages of dementia, one is apt to be misled by such facades in earlier stages of the illness. As Henry Brosin[8] pointed out:

> Injury to the cerebral cortex means injury also to the ego functions, not only mechanically but psychologically, for the cerebral functions are highly valued by man, and any diminution in their efficacy causes apprehension and concern, which in turn arouse defensive measures to protect the total organism from pain and harm. An organism uncertain of its spatial-temporal-social relations (disturbance of the comprehension of the environment), as brain-damaged cases are, is much more vulnerable to suffering than the normal person, even though much of the basic core of the ego be intact—as it so often is.

It is easy for the physician to be deluded into believing there is an absence of pain and vulnerability to suffering in the demented patient who so blatantly denies his losses and limitations. At a deeper level of realization, however, we cannot conceive the disintegration of the mind as anything other than an agonizing process for the affected individual. The denials and evasions employed by the demented person to hide his failures[21] can then be seen as naive and feeble defense mechanisms, and the physician can no longer hide from himself the inevitable pain of mental disintegration.

The needs of the family must also not be ignored. "An illness of this kind affects others besides those who suffer from it, and the idea that a loved person—or oneself for that matter—might be transformed into something alien is disquieting. Pain and incapacity and disfigurement can be faced with fortitude, but the sight of a disease which seems to rot the self is hard to bear."[4] Close consultation with the family is needed not only to provide for their needs but because they often possess that intimate knowledge of the patient's premorbid personality which is essential for his optimal care.

The care of the demented patient can be formulated quite simply and easily; its execution, however, presents formidable difficulties. In essence, the patient's care is based upon thorough assessment of his liabilities (lost functions) and assets (preserved functions), physical and psychological, coupled with a knowledge of his premorbid personality characteristics. Treatment is aimed at: (1) restitution of those lost functions which are susceptible to restitution; (2) reduction of the patient's need to employ those functions that have been lost; and (3) maximal utilization of residual functions. The value of such an approach has been proved by Sklar and O'Neill[34] and by others before them.

Restitution of Lost Functions

This aims predominantly at correction of medical and physical limitations. Many demented patients are debilitated and cachectic through neglect of physical ailments, nutritional needs, and exercise requirements. It is unwise to expect other measures to effect significant improvement unless the patient is in the best possible physical condition. Prompt and thorough treatment of medical disorders is, if anything, more important in the demented patient than in the one not so affected. The vulnerability of the diseased brain to fever, infection, and toxins is well recognized but often poorly recalled. The nutritional needs of the patient may be hard to satisfy because of his inattention and lack of concern, with resulting vitamin deficiencies and inanition. Continuous efforts to assure an adequate and judicious dietary intake are essential. Physiotherapy can promote restitution of lost motor function (and prevent its loss in ambulatory patients). Since the physical, psychiatric, and social problems of the bed- or chair-ridden patient with dementia are infinitely more formidable than those faced by the ambulatory patient, every effort should be made to preserve and promote motility.

Reduction of the Patient's Need for Functions That Have Been Lost

An accurate assessment of what functions have been irretrievably lost is essential. The pressures suffered by the demented patient who battles to perform impossible tasks or valiantly struggles to hide his failures are apparent to all observers. Often, at least up to the terminal phases of the disorder, the patient is helpless to give up the fight. Thus Katz, Neal, and Simon[21] have recorded the multiple defenses used by demented patients to avoid acquiescing to failure, to avoid admitting, "I don't know." They also emphasize how demands for task performance are stressful and how immediate stress is often a determinant of symptomatology. Whereas stress in the intact individual may enhance the ego, stress in the demented patient may lead to ego disintegration.

This has been elegantly described by one author writing of her father's illness.[4] Although she knew her father to have failing mental powers, she unwisely agreed to accompany him to a foreign resort. There the foreign language and unfamiliar surroundings markedly accentuated his bewilderment and his anxiety.

He was still potentially rational. His delusions were not determined by a warped mental outlook, but were a reasonable attempt to make sense out of what was subjectively a hopelessly confusing situation. In days gone by I had learned to follow his train of thought intuitively, and I could still keep close to him in spite of his difficulty with speech. I found that if I got him away from other people and steered his mind to topics which he had handled with ease in the past he became rational quite quickly. I sometimes led him into long and interesting discussions on subjects which he knew and cared about, and when he got the sense of being on familiar ground, where he could still tread firmly, the black cloud of depression lifted and he became his old self. As soon as he returned to the strain of new and unfamiliar situations he relapsed.

Using such techniques she was able to maintain some self-control in her father until World War II intervened, providing a stress that she was powerless to control. "Faced with a threat which involved his own country and all that was dear to him, my father let go his last faint hold on reason . . . ."

Environmental manipulation can be used to maintain calm and nontaxing surroundings, arranging things insofar as is possible so that the patient does not have to confront his inadequacies. Often ingenious techniques may be employed to achieve this objective. One patient, for example, who was disoriented in space but still able to read, was greatly calmed by messages appropriately placed by her family over the house, saying, "You're in your bedroom," "You're in your parlor," and similar notes.[1]

Utilization of Residual Functions

For the demented individual to utilize his remaining functions fully, the physician must assume dual roles: (1) as personal physician to the individual patient; (2) as organizer of health care delivery by various individuals and agencies.

One of his functions as personal physician to the individual patient is to prescribe medications for the relief of symptoms. In the demented patient, medications may be employed to: (1) relieve anxiety, (2) improve mood, (3) reduce paranoid symptoms, and (4) improve sleep. Treatment is employed here for symptoms arising as a result of organic brain disease; symptomatic results are not as good as when psychotropic agents are employed in the functional psychiatric disorders. At times, however, medications may be remarkably effective, and they certainly should be tried.

Two points concerning drug treatment in organic dementias should be underscored: (1) Sedatives are poorly tolerated in the presence of structural brain disease; therefore, barbiturates and like medications should be avoided. (2) The damaged central nervous system may be exquisitely sensitive to psychotropic agents; thus treatment should be begun with doses quite small in comparison to those employed in functional brain disorders.[10]

For relief of nonpsychotic anxiety, chlordiazepoxide (Librium), 5 mg. twice daily, or diazepam (Valium), 2 mg. twice daily, may prove useful. The dosage may be raised to achieve better symptom relief, but only slowly, cautiously, and under close medical supervision. These medications tend to lose their effectiveness with continued use. For depression, amitriptyline (Elavil), nortriptyline (Aventyl), and imipramine (Tofranil) may be employed. In patients with dementia plus depression, starting dosage should probably be no more than

10 mg. three or four times daily for any of these antidepressant medications. As with the minor tranquilizers the dosage can be raised, but only under close supervision. For paranoid symptoms, chlorpromazine (Thorazine) or thioridazine (Mellaril), 25 mg. three or four times daily, or haloperidol (Haldol), 0.5 mg. two or three times daily, should be tried. Again, doses may be adjusted upward with close supervision. In patients with insomnia, drugs with minimal sedative effects should be employed to help achieve sleep. Promethazine hydrochloride (Phenergan), 25 to 50 mg. at bedtime, or chlorpromazine (Thorazine), 50 mg. at bedtime, is often effective. For the acutely disturbed patient, chlorpromazine, 25 mg. intramuscularly, is the drug of choice.

All of the medications have undesirable central nervous system effects that must be looked for closely. In addition, the phenothiazines often precipitate postural hypotension, a particularly unfortunate side-effect in the aged group often being treated for dementia.

Whether it is called providing supportive psychotherapy or performing the physician's role, the physician furnishes another essential service to the patient.

> The foreign doctor came and went again, leaving a sedative which was unfortunately a proprietary brand with the contents printed outside the container. My father feared we were intent on drugging him for some nefarious purpose, and he would not touch it. He had, however, recognized the doctor for what he was, and the visit sobered him a little. Even that much relief was something to be thankful for...[4]

The physician's presence alone may thus be important. He supports and encourages the patient to develop his interests, to continue social activities, to partake in group activities, to exercise, to be productive in ways in which he can be appreciated by others as long as is possible.[10, 34] He allows the patient to ventilate feelings of anger, rejection, fear, and hurt—accepting them, appreciating them, and thus "detoxifying" them. The role of the physician's expectations in both symptom production and in symptom relief has never been fully explored in these situations, but it is probably of great importance.[13, 23]

The second responsibility of the physician is to organize the various health professionals and nonprofessionals who partake in the patient's care so that the most satisfactory treatment possible results. This may involve weaving together the ministrations of the physician, nurse, social worker, occupational therapist, recreational therapist, physiotherapist, and the family — and each role may be crucial. For example, Sklar and O'Neill[34] have observed that little can be accomplished by psychiatric treatment "in the absence of successful solution of the patient's social problem." The social problem cannot be solved of course without the cooperation of the family, and others. The melding of these various individuals to create a successful treatment program is difficult even in the hospital. Outside the in-patient setting, the problems of creating such a treatment program are staggering but worthy of our efforts.

These three avenues constitute the essential approaches to the symptomatic treatment of dementia. None aims directly to improve function of disease neurons; rather the aims are to permit the still functioning neurons to perform optimally. Recently a number of therapeutic measures have been reported to improve brain function per se, and their widespread use has been advocated. We face a serious problem in evaluation of these reports. The use of the therapeutic measures advocated above has resulted in rather striking clinical improvement in groups of patients[34] as has the use of group activities to provide sensory stimulation[7] and the use of placebos.[29] Will other measures enhance our results? The difficulties of evaluating the effects of drugs on cerebral function have already been detailed by Appel and Festoff.[5] They conclude that no drug presently available has been proved of value in improving cerebral function in the demented patient, though there are suggestions that one or two chemicals may improve performance secondary to their general stimulant effects. They also raise the possibility that stimulation of the failing neuron might hasten its demise, though they carefully point out there is no specific evidence of this at present. There is presently available no medication that will predictably improve cerebral function in the demented patient; further, the benefits or desirability of use of the stimulant drugs is unconvincing. This is nevertheless an important area of investigation that should not be abandoned merely because of past failures.

Ventriculoatrial shunting has recently been reported valuable in the treatment of degenerative brain disease.[32] In some of the cases reported, improvement was spectacular. The field of dementia is, however, strewn with discarded remedies, successfully employed for a while by one individual but lacking in consistency of responses or ineffective in the hands of others. Because of the notorious difficulty in evaluating treatment of dementia, and because the studies have not been replicated, judgment of the efficacy of shunting procedures in cerebral degeneration (when it is not due to spinal fluid malabsorption) must be withheld.

CONCLUSION

In many ways, dementia can be regarded as a vast lacuna in our neuropsychiatric knowledge, unfulfilling in its study because so much is unknown and so little understood. Were the condition rare, we might take comfort in devoting our efforts to more pressing problems. Unfortunately dementia is common and becoming more so. The pain and suffering it causes patients and their families are great, as are the frustration and discouragement it provokes in their physicians. The proper care of the demented patient requires uncommon time, effort, and devotion by the physician and makes uncommon demands upon the family and community resources. There is little question that these unfortunate individuals do not now generally receive the best care possible, even allowing that the best care possible falls short of our goals. Perhaps we should be reminded, as was another physician by the husband of a woman with irreversible brain damage, "Doctor—you should have seen her as the wonderful person she is."[18]

REFERENCES

1. ACKNER, B.: Personal communication.

2. ALPERS, B. J., FORSTER, F. M., AND HERBUT, P. A.: *Retinal, cerebral and systemic arteriosclerosis; a histopathologic study.* Arch. Neurol. Psychiat. 60:440, 1948.

3. AMERICAN PSYCHIATRIC ASSOCIATION: *Diagnostic and Statistical Manual of Mental Disorders,* ed. 2. American Psychiatric Association, Washington, D. C., 1968.

4. ANONYMOUS AUTHOR: *Death of a mind: A study of disintegration.* Lancet 1:1012, 1950.

5. APPEL, S. H., AND FESTOFF, B. W.: Biochemical dysfunction and dementia, in Wells, C. E. (ed.) : *Dementia.* F. A. Davis Co., Philadelphia, 1971, Chap. 8.

6. BENNETT, J. E., HASENCLEVER, H. F., AND TYNES, B. S.: *Detection of cryptococcal polysaccharide in serum and spinal fluid: Value in diagnosis and prognosis.* Trans. Assn. Amer. Phys. 77:145, 1964.

7. BOWER, H. M.: *Sensory stimulation and the treatment of senile dementia.* Med. J. Australia 1:1113, 1967.

8. BROSIN, H. W.: Contributions of psychoanalysis to the study of organic cerebral disorders, in Alexander, F., and Ross, H., (eds.) : *Dynamic Psychiatry.* University of Chicago Press, Chicago, 1952, pp. 211-254.

9. BUCHWALD, J.: 'Just an Old Crock' (Editorial). Psychiatric News 4:2, 1969.

10. BUSSE, E. W.: Psychoneurotic reactions and defense mechanisms in the aged, in Hoch, P. H., and Zubin, J. (eds.) : *Psychopathology of Aging.* American Psychopathological Association Proceedings, 1960, pp. 274-284.

11. BUSSE, E. W., AND PFEIFFER, E.: Functional psychiatric disorders in old age, in Busse, E. W., and Pfeiffer, E. (eds.) : *Bahavior and Adaptation in Late Life.* Little, Brown and Company, Boston, 1969, pp. 183-235.

12. BUTLER, W. T., ALLING, D. W., SPICKARD, A., AND UTZ, J. P.: *Diagnostic and prognostic value of clinical and laboratory findings in cryptococcal meningitis.* New Eng. J. Med. 270:59, 1964.

13. CAMERON, D. E.: Discussion of paper by Lorge, I.[23] Res. Publ. Assn. Res. Nerv. Ment. Dis. 35:57, 1956.

14. FISHER, C. M.: *Dementia in cerebral vascular disease.* Trans. Sixth Conf. on Cerebral Vascular Diseases. Grune & Stratton, Inc., New York, 1968, pp. 232-236.

15. GORDON, N. A., AND VEDDER, D. K.: *Serologic tests in diagnosis and prognosis of cryptococcosis.* J.A.M.A. 197:961, 1966.

16. GREEN, M. A., STEVENSON, L. D., FONSECA, J. E., AND WORTIS, S. B.: *Cerebral biopsy in patients with presenile dementia.* Dis. Nerv. Syst. 13:303, 1952.

17. HAASE, G. R.: Diseases presenting as dementia, in Wells, C. E. (ed.) : *Dementia.* F. A. Davis Co., Philadelphia, 1971, Chap. 10.

18. HORENSTEIN, S.: Amnestic, agnosic, apractic, and aphasic features in dementing illness, in Wells, C. E. (ed.) : *Dementia*, F. A. Davis Co., Philadelphia, 1971, Chap. 3.

19. HORENSTEIN, S.: The clinical use of psychological testing in dementia, in Wells, C. E. (ed.) : *Dementia*. F. A. Davis Co., Philadelphia, 1971, Chap. 4.

20. KAPLAN, E. A.: Personal communication, 1970.

21. KATZ, L., NEAL, M. W., AND SIMON, A.: Observations of psychic mechanisms in organic psychoses of the aged, in Hoch, P. H., and Zubin, J., (eds.) : *Psychopathology of Aging*. American Psychopathological Association Proceedings, 1960, pp. 160-181.

22. LEWIS, A.: *Amnesic syndromes. The psychopathological aspects*. Proc. Roy. Soc. Med. 54:955, 1961.

23. LORGE, I.: *Aging and intelligence*. Res. Publ. Assn. Nerv. Ment. Dis. 35:46, 1956.

24. McDOWELL, F., AND WOLFF, H. G.: *Handbook of Neurological Diagnostic Methods*. The Williams & Wilkins Co., Baltimore, 1960.

25. McDOWELL, F.: Personal communication, 1970.

26. MEACHAM, W. F., AND YOUNG, A. B.: Radiological procedures in the diagnosis of dementia, in Wells, C. E. (ed.): *Dementia*. F. A. Davis Co., Philadelphia, 1971, Chap. 6.

27. MERRITT, H. H., ADAMS, R. D., AND SOLOMON, H. C.: *Neurosyphilis*, Oxford University Press, Inc., New York, 1946.

28. NICHOLAS, L., AND LENTZ, J. W.: *Diagnosis of syphilis in the geriatric patient*. Geriatrics 23:169, 1968.

29. NODINE, J. H., SHULKIN, M. W., SLAP, J. W., LEVINE, M., AND FREIBERG, K.: *A double-blind study of the effect of ribonucleic acid in senile brain disease*. Amer. J. Psychiat. 123:1257, 1967.

30. PAULSON, G. W.: The neurological examination in dementia, in Wells, C. E. (ed.) : *Dementia*. F. A. Davis Co., Philadelphia, 1971, Chap. 2.

31. ROTH, M.: *The natural history of mental disorder in old age*. J. Ment. Sci. 101:281, 1955.

32. SALMON, J. H., AND ARMITAGE, J. L.: *Surgical treatment of hydrocephalus ex vacuo. Ventriculoatrial shunt for degenerative brain disease*. Neurology 18:1223, 1968.

33. SIM, M., TURNER, E., AND SMITH, W. T.: *Cerebral biopsy in the investigation of presenile dementia. I. Clinical aspects*. Brit. J. Psychiat. 112:119, 1966.

34. SKLAR, J., AND O'NEILL, F. J.: Experiments with intensive treatment in a geriatric ward, in Hoch, P. H., and Zubin, J., (eds.) : *Psychopathology of Aging*. American Psychopathological Association Proceedings, 1960, pp. 266-273.

35. SMITH, J. L.: *Spirochetes in Late Seronegative Syphilis, Penicillin Notwithstanding*. Charles C Thomas, Publisher, Springfield, Ill., 1969.

36. SMITH, J. L., SINGER, J. A., MOORE, M. B., AND YOBS, A.: *Seronegative ocular and neurosyphilis.* Amer. J. Ophthal. 59:753, 1965.

37. TORACK, R. M.: *Ultrastructural and histochemical studies in a case of progressive dementia and its relationship to protein metabolism.* Amer. J. Path. 49:77, 1966.

38. WANG, H. S., AND BUSSE, E. W.: Dementia in old age, in Wells, C. E. (ed.): *Dementia.* F. A. Davis Co., Philadelphia, 1971, Chap. 9.

39. WELLS, C. E.: The symptoms and behavioral manifestations of dementia, in Wells, C. E. (ed.): *Dementia.* F. A. Davis Co., Philadelphia, 1971, Chap. 1.

40. WELLS, C. E.: Unpublished observations.

41. WHYBROW, P. C., PRANGE, A. J., JR., AND TREADWAY, C. R.: *Mental changes accompanying thryroid gland dysfunction.* Arch. Gen. Psychiat. 20:48, 1969.

Index